CW01636124

AIDS, CANCER AND ARTHRITIS

A NEW PERSPECTIVE

PHYLLIS EVELYN PEASE D.Sc. Ph.D.

Former Senior Lecturer in Medical Microbiology
University of Birmingham, United Kingdom

ISBN 0-9550567-0-5

043616

CONTENTS

PAGE

FOREWORD iii
by Sir David Smith FRS

PREFACE v

CHAPTER 1 10
Bacteria as a Biological Group

CHAPTER 2 23
The Mycoplasmas

CHAPTER 3 39
Bacterial Elements as Crypto-infective Agents in Human Blood

CHAPTER 4 47
Infection with Alien DNA - the Extreme Case of Infectious Aetiology

CHAPTER 5 57
Retroviruses as Genetic Engineers

CHAPTER 6 73
Immunological Aspects

CHAPTER 7 85
The Malignancies

CHAPTER 8 111
AIDS

CHAPTER 9 137
AIDS and other Immunopathologies

AFTERWORD 163

GLOSSARY 173

APPENDIX 1 178
Brief notes on some Autoimmune Diseases

APPENDIX 2 181
Is Bovine Spongiform Encephalopathy (BSE) an Autoimmune Disease?

ACKNOWLEDGEMENTS 183

FOREWORD

I met Phyllis Pease at a series of interdisciplinary conferences. These aimed to bring together a wide diversity of biological scientists with a common interest in the cell as an environment both for microorganisms and for DNA derived from other cells and organisms. The initial stimulus for these conferences was the developing acceptance in the late 1970s and early 1980s that during the evolution of the modern eukaryotic cell, one or more of its organelles had resulted from the early acquisition of microorganisms at some stage in the Precambrian era.

It had taken some years for this concept of cell evolution to gain credence. Indeed, when the American biologist, Lynn Margulis, first advocated in 1969 that mitochondria had evolved from symbiotic aerobic bacteria, the great majority of cell scientists strongly disagreed with her. Some of their comments were quite derisory, and almost all funding agencies peremptorily refused her applications for research grants on the topic. In 1970, when I referred to Lynn's ideas in a lecture to first year university students, I was reprimanded by a senior colleague for mentioning 'such rubbish'. However, at that time, it had been universally believed for a century or more that the eukaryotic cell had evolved from a single prokaryotic cell simply by way of intracellular differentiation and compartmentalisation. It was unthinkable then that the DNA of mitochondria could have had any other derivation than from the cell nucleus.

Nowadays, of course, the symbiotic origin of mitochondria and certain other cellular bodies is taken for granted by almost all cell biologists. The universality of the genetic code, and the basic similarity in mechanisms of protein synthesis between widely different organisms, make it easy to accept that the nucleus can control the growth and division of these ancestrally free-living bodies as well as accepting the transfer of some DNA from them. Indeed, the cell can be an environment for just fragments of DNA from other cells, whether of its own species or different species. It is well known that modern techniques of genetic engineering enable some genes to be transferred between widely different kinds of organism (such as between jellyfish and plants). It is reasonable to assume that various forms of 'natural' genetic engineering must have occurred widely throughout evolution - and are still occurring today.

It was at one of these interdisciplinary conferences in 1989 that I heard Phyllis - a medical microbiologist - present a fascinating paper. She showed that the bacteria which cause tumours (such as crown gall) or root nodules on legumes can also be commonly isolated from humans. It is known that in crown gall, the bacterial tumour-inducing agent is actually borne on a plasmid, part of whose DNA may have been originally acquired from another plant. While this certainly did not indicate that these particular bacteria can cause human cancer, it did shed light on a possible role of foreign DNA carried by bacteria in human and other animal diseases. Sadly, these avenues have received little exploration in modern medicine, and in general, the willingness to explore ideas and techniques generated by such cross-disciplinary endeavours is uncommon. The situation of research into autoimmune diseases in general, and AIDS in particular, described in this book presents a sad example of this. Those of us like myself who are distant from AIDS research have derived our knowledge of it from popular science journals. We are led to believe there is incontestable, cast-iron proof that AIDS is caused by HIV. We naturally assume that the cell preparations used in experiments have been demonstrated to be free of contaminants by the usual rigorous tests for microbiological purity - and especially by electron microscopy. We take it for granted that the possibility that infective particles other than HIV are the causal agents has been ruled out by exhaustive, rigorously conducted experiments.

It is therefore an eye-opener to read from this book that such evidence that AIDS is solely caused by HIV does not exist, and that research into autoimmune diseases in general leaves much to be desired. The absolute purity of cell preparations used in many experiments is to be seriously questioned. Koch's postulates have not been proven. The straightforward, dispassionate analysis in this book of the experimental techniques used and the quality of the evidence they generate gives important grounds for concern, especially given the seriousness of the world-wide AIDS epidemic, and the huge investment in research based on the assumption that there is no other possible cause of AIDS than HIV.

It is not uncommon for those whose views, however justified, which go against the grain of current scientific beliefs to be ignored or even derided. Unfortunately, Lynn Margulis' experience in the early 1970s is but one of many examples of this. Sadly, there have also been recent examples of ostracism of those who dare to question whether HIV is the causal agent of AIDS. This particular book is not about 'beliefs', but about critical, careful analysis of the experimental techniques that are used. It reveals the lack of any determined pursuit of potentially valuable lines of investigation suggested either by deficiencies in these techniques, or by related situations in organisms other than human beings.

I found it both a stimulating and a very salutary book to read - especially at a time when public scepticism about the outcomes of certain types of scientific research has reached a worrying level. It is very important that the critical analyses made in this book are widely read.

David Smith

Sir David Smith FRS
Founder Member of the International Society of Endocytobiology
Principal of Edinburgh University 1989-1994
Head of the largest graduate college (Wolfson) Oxford University 1994-2000
Currently government advisor on environmental concerns

PREFACE

You've got to use an approach you're completely sure of. I mean literally, that whenever there is confusion or doubt in your mind, the first thing to do is to recover your bearings. Any guide or explorer will tell you that. When they realise they are lost, or they've taken the wrong road, they won't take a short cut through the forest, nor do they rely on their instincts to set them back to the right direction. What they do is to go back carefully over the whole road until they've found their starting point, or the point at which they took the wrong turn.

Alfred Hitchcock (1986)*

I have previously** suggested that a natural genetic engineering (NGE) mechanism involving bacterial vectors could account for certain human diseases which seem to be associated with infective agents but not in the conventional way. There are many such diseases, including rheumatic, nephritic and haemolytic disorders and recently the advent of the AIDS epidemic has focussed attention on them. The reason for this is that AIDS patients are particularly prone to develop auto-antibodies and in this respect AIDS can be regarded as belonging to this group of immunopathologies, which are usually referred to as the autoimmune diseases. It has also become apparent in the intervening years that malignant diseases may also fall into the same category.

My suggestion concerning the autoimmunities was that bacteria could act as carriers of DNA and transport it into the nuclei of human cells; that if colonisation were successful, disease might follow because the infected cell would have different characteristics and be recognised as foreign by the host's immune system. Thus this system would bring about an attack on what in reality are the body's own cells, and disease would follow.

In this second book I have tried to explain that this bacterial/vector role for the transportation of DNA from one source into the DNA of a related human or animal is still a viable hypothesis to explain what might be legitimately be called the clonal diseases of man and some animals. These include the malignancies and the autoimmunities, possibly including AIDS. In the presentation of this view it has been necessary to address the supposed role of retroviruses in these disorders and a study of retrovirology within a much wider biological context than has hitherto been customary has led me to believe that the claims that they are disease-causing agents are not based on sound foundations..

Here I have taken the view that a wrong turning was taken in 1970, which has not only impeded progress in cancer research but has led to the retrovirus/HIV equals AIDS concept, which according to a number of investigators is a total misconception. Their doubts are basically concerned with the haste with which certain valid important observations were adopted by the retroviral cause without due cognisance being taken of alternative explanations and that this state of affairs has been very considerably compounded by the use of uncontrolled techniques.

The latter seem to have occurred because biochemists, who in my experience usually have a poor understanding of microorganisms as living creatures and have a tendency to regard bacteria as laboratory tools - for example, as bags of enzymes or as culture media for the propagation of designer plasmids - and believe that biochemical techniques are all that is necessary for the identification and isolation of viruses. Frequently, medically trained individuals regard micro-organisms as basically potential pathogens and all too often, where AIDS research is concerned, they have adopted the same techniques employed by the biochemists.

The result of this simplistic approach is that it has been accompanied by the virtual abandonment of that *sine qua non* for a properly trained microbiologist, the microscope, and in the case of filterable forms of bacteria and viruses this means the electron-microscope. Without these aids and the controls that they offer, it has become apparent that what have passed as preparations of pure virions have in fact been contaminated not only with filterable forms of bacteria but also with cellular materials derived from the tissue-cultures in which the viruses have been cultured.

Returning to the bacterial-vector path - experimental support for the notion of bacteria acting as vectors for disease-causing DNA followed shortly after my earlier publication and came from plant biologists who discovered the phenomenon in the causation of plant cancer. The bacterium involved is *Agrobacterium tumefaciens*, which causes cancer only when it is itself infected with a plasmid, part of which causes tumours. It is now understood that the alien DNA in question is associated with growth control mechanisms, and that on colonisation of the plant host nucleus, the intruding DNA interferes with the normal control mechanisms of the host cells, resulting in excess cellular proliferation and by a progressive process leads eventually to full malignancy.

Shortly before this natural genetic engineering *modus operandi* as a cause of disease was worked out there was renewed interest in the possibility that a similar *Agrobacterium*-like bacterium might have a parallel role in human cancer and in late 1969 a meeting was held by the New York Academy of Sciences at which this was the main topic of discussion. It was also suggested at this meeting that the tumour viruses responsible for cancer causation in birds and mammals (re-named retroviruses a few months later) might actually be filterable forms of bacteria.

Six years later it was discovered that the cancer-causing properties of these tumour-causing agents are due to their ability to act as vectors for alien DNA that is capable of interfering with the growth control mechanisms of the infected host. The source of the alien DNA in these cases is in the DNA of another host and is nothing to do with the virus-like agent *per se*. This indicates that the underlying mechanism for cancer causation is fundamentally the same for plants and higher eukaryotes.

From a biological point of view, the malignancies are considerably easier to investigate than the immunopathologies because they are disorders of multicellular organisms in which, by definition there is a built-in potential for individual cell/cells to escape from the control mechanisms that maintain the *status quo*. Thus models, particularly the plant cancer one capable of supplying information relevant to the condition in humans, are available. In the case of auto-immune diseases the difficulty lies in the fact that these are essentially the disorders of higher animals that have developed an immune system and no simple model can therefore exist.

However, since my earlier publication two very important advances have been made in this area. One is the elucidation of the HLA (human leukocyte antigen system - the antigens that determine the human self) and the second related one is the discovery that some HLA types are associated with particular diseases. These developments make it possible to envisage that the putative invasive DNA in the immunological disorders encodes for immune-regulating proteins rather than the growth regulating ones that are characteristic of the invading DNA in the malignancies.

In my presentation of the case for bacterial vectors having a vital role as DNA vectors in human clonal diseases I have made a great deal of use of microscopic, particularly electron-microscopic, images, several of which are my own preparations, to demonstrate both the morphology of sub-cellular elements of bacteria including mycoplasmas, an area that is not widely known, as well as to indicate that failure to use these tools has led to serious errors of interpretation and the *impasse* that AIDS research in particular has now reached. As far as references are concerned, I have tried to make the text comprehensible to scientists in other disciplines as well as interested laymen, at the same time providing enough references for specialists to follow up should they wish to do so.

Phyllis Pease
Montjoie-en-Couserans

* Alfred Hitchcock was talking about the expensive failure, 'Under Capricorn'.
Truffaut, F. (1984) Hitchcock by Truffaut; The definitive study.
Paladin Grafton Books London, Glasgow, Sydney Auckland.

** Pease P. E. (1965) L-Forms, Episomes and Autoimmune Disease.
E &S Livingston Ltd, Edinburgh and London

CHAPTER ONE

BACTERIA AS A BIOLOGICAL GROUP

'Young woman, can you imagine any living species, and particularly so easily destructible (sic) ones as bacteria, that would be able to survive the environmental changes of moisture and temperature and the vicissitudes of life if they did not have a life-cycle?'

'These forms of bacteria are ubiquitous. They survive in soils, they are carried by seed and are transmitted by other parasites, and if you plant pathologists do not soon heed them the day may come when humanity is without daily bread.'

Beijerink (1925)

'There are three main habitats for living organisms, land, water and other living organisms'

D.C. Smith (1979)

INTRODUCTION 12

THE CYTOLOGY AND LIFE-HISTORY OF BACTERIA 13

PARASITES AND GENETICS OF BACTERIA 16

POSSIBLE RELATION OF BACTERIAL PARASITES TO HUMAN IMMUNOPATHOLOGIES AND MALIGNANCIES 18

SUMMARY 19

INTRODUCTION

Generally speaking, bacteria are seen as disease causing organisms, biochemical agents, agricultural agents and occasionally as useful laboratory agents, e.g. for the testing of medical products for sterility. More recently, their ability to act as vectors (carriers) of DNA from other unrelated species, including humans, has become widely known in the context of genetic engineering (GE).

However, in contrast to the bacteria that are 'tamed' for these various purposes in the laboratory, they are, if left to their own devices, capable of behaving as living creatures in their own right and have developed a considerable range of tactics for their survival. Moreover, bacteria in the wild may also carry alien DNA, which may cause damage, including cancer, in other living creatures. This process is described as natural genetic engineering (NGE). In fact it was the study of the natural phenomenon that led to its exploitation in the laboratory for the purposes of the improvement of crops and the development of certain medical procedures such as gene therapy.

Bacteria are almost always described as unicellular even in the scientific press and indeed the most famous bacterium, *Escherichia coli*, is unicellular, but the multicellularity characteristic of many bacteria is obscured by the standard techniques of heat-fixation and staining methods - especially the gram stain - employed in clinical diagnostic laboratories. The use of these methods for the original intention of identifying disease-causing bacteria served this purpose very well, but they are totally unsuitable for the investigation of the true morphology and cytology of the bacteria. In spite of this, most students have grown up with the notion that heat-fixation followed by gram-staining gives a true picture of the bacteria, and gram-positivity or negativity is almost always recorded in species descriptions.

More gentle techniques have been developed in order to demonstrate the true nature of the organisms in the light-microscope. These avoid heat-fixation and drying, and it has become apparent that there is a good case for regarding bacteria as living cells with the same structure and function as other living cells. These types of studies were initially an esoteric pursuit, which enjoyed a burst of popularity in the thirties, and then again in the fifties and sixties with the development of the transmission and scanning electron microscopes and techniques for ultra-sectioning.

Since the sixties however, the status of bacteria as creatures with lives of their own, so to speak, has tended to be disregarded. As a result, their potential to cause problems as troublesome contaminants causing misleading, even disastrous, results in scientific experiments has been obscured. The mycoplasmas, which are a group of bacteria that lack a cell and are discussed in the next chapter, have been especially notorious in this respect due to their troublesome habit of contaminating tissue cultures in which viruses are cultured, thus giving rise to errors of interpretation. This hazard was first recognised in the late fifties and re-surfaced in the eighties to plague AIDS research in particular. Unfortunately, this fact has been misunderstood or ignored by almost all AIDS investigators, and has led to a great deal of misinformation, which still persists today. This aspect of bacteria in AIDS research in particular is discussed at length in the following chapters.

In the meantime it is the purpose of this chapter to examine bacteria as a biological group of organisms, many of which are capable of living in the three habitats of 'land, water and other living creatures'. In these habitats, bacteria behave differently from the way they do when cultured artificially in the laboratory, and it is from this perspective that the organisms need to be viewed in order to understand how they can act as agents in the transport of potentially disease-causing DNA in humans.

THE CYTOLOGY AND LIFE-HISTORY OF BACTERIA

The use of more gentle techniques for the examination of bacteria enabled the cell-walls and nuclei to be demonstrated in the light microscope (Figs 1.1a -1.1f), and the development of techniques of ultra-sectioning for electron-microscopy confirmed and enhanced these studies. As is the case with other biological groups, bacteria may possess a variety of structures such as flagella; fimbriae or pili; capsules and spores.

Flagella, the organs of motility, which can be detected by direct microscopic viewing of the motility of the bacteria in fluid medium and which can also be very easily demonstrated in the electron microscope and whose arrangement *i.e.* whether at the poles (bipolar or monopolar) or all round the bacteria (peritrichous) and whose numbers sometimes can be aids to identification; capsules, which are surface layers of mucoid or gelatinous materials, can also be useful in bacterial identification.

Fimbriae or pili which bear some superficial resemblance to flagella but are shorter and straight and are not concerned with motility. Some, the somatic ones, contribute to the pathogenicity of bacteria in as much as they enable them to adhere to various specific surfaces whereas others have a sexual function (see below).

Some bacteria produce spores which are resistant to conditions harmful to vegetative bacteria, *e.g.* high temperatures and disinfectants and other antibacterial agents. The morphology of spores and their position on the bacteria can aid identification, the classic case being the characteristic drumstick spores of *Clostridium tetani* (Fig. 1.1f) Spore formation in effect represents one of the simpler forms of a bacterial life-cycle, in which vegetative bacteria produce resistant spores which do not divide in this form, but which, when conditions are favourable, germinate and give rise to the vegetative forms directly.

The possession of such life-cycles, to a greater or lesser extent, is an example of yet another way in which bacteria resemble other biological groups, and, as is common among other biological groups, the phylogeny of certain types of bacteria can be determined by reference to their life-cycles.

Fig. 1.1 The Cytology of Bacteria

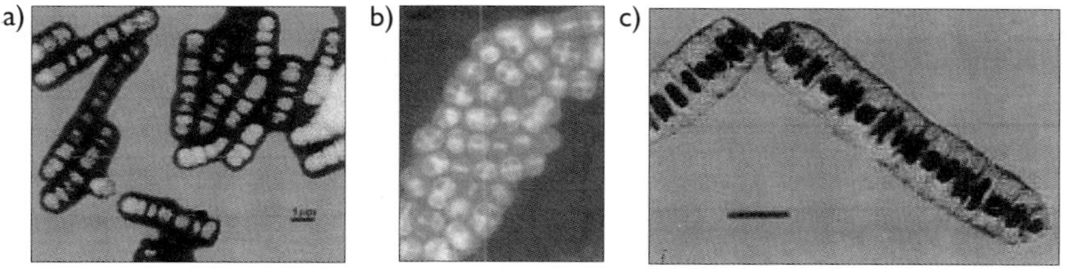

a) Caryophanon - a large bacterium showing cell-walls
b) *Staphylococcus aureus* showing cell-walls
c) Oscillospira- another bacterium showing nuclei

d) 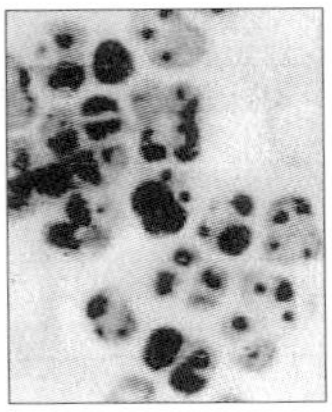 e) 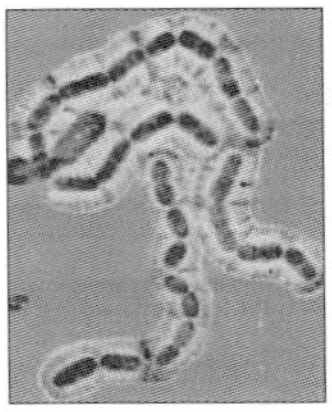 f) 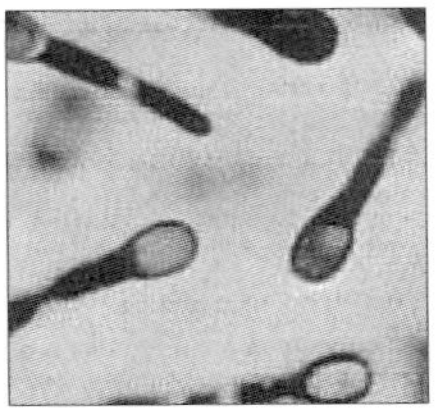

d) *Aerobacter aerogenes* showing nuclei
e) *Bacillus spp.* showing capsules around the chain of bacteria
f) Terminal bacterial spores. Those of *C.tetani* are more rounded

Other life-cycles more complicated than the simple 'spore to bacterium and back', exist in bacteria, and much of the basic information necessary for the understanding of them and their importance to the NGE concept of disease can be gained by reference to those studied in our laboratory. These include *Spirillum, Pseudomonas, Yersinia, Rhizobium* and *Agrobacterium*.

Spirilla, which are aquatic bacteria, are useful for the demonstration of a bacterial life-cycle because they are relatively large organisms and undergo the cycle readily and spontaneously in initial enrichment cultures and subsequently in young cultures established in the laboratory on nutrient agar (Pease 1956).

Their life-cycles can be demonstrated by stained impression preparations and electron-microscopy. Impression preparations are made by cutting a portion of agar upon which the colonies of interest are growing, inverting it onto a microscope slide, applying a slight amount of pressure and then fixing it, e.g. picric acid. The agar block is then removed leaving the impression on the slide so that it can be stained.

Fig. 1.2 Impression Preparations of *Spirillum Serpens* Showing Stages in its Life-cycle

a) 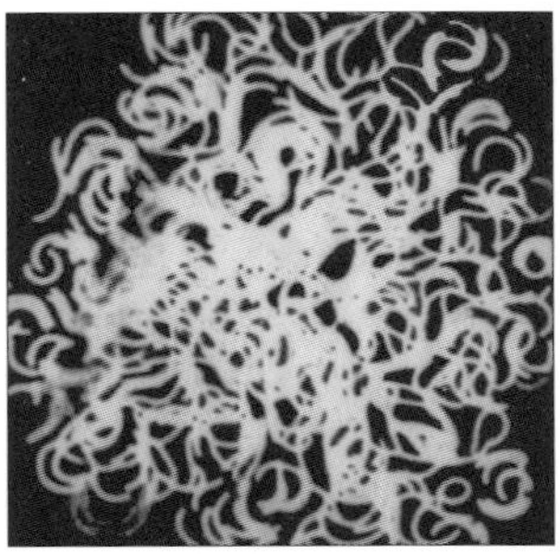 b) 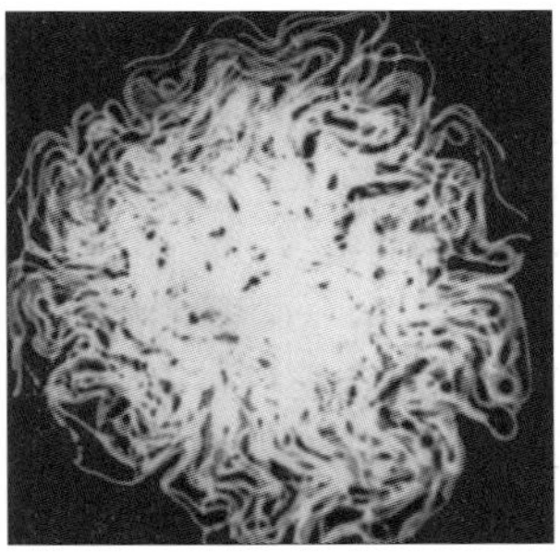 c) 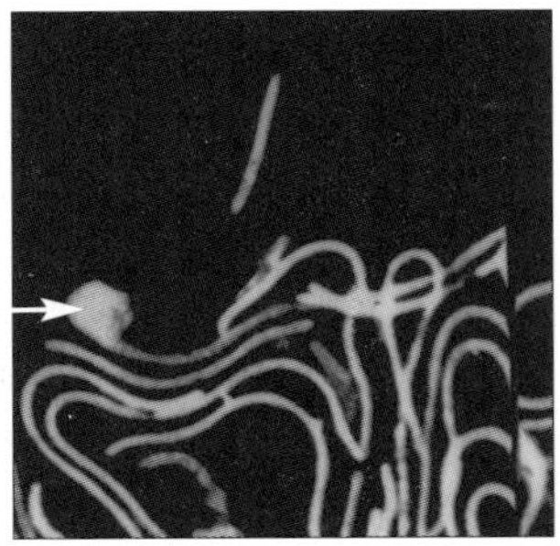

d) 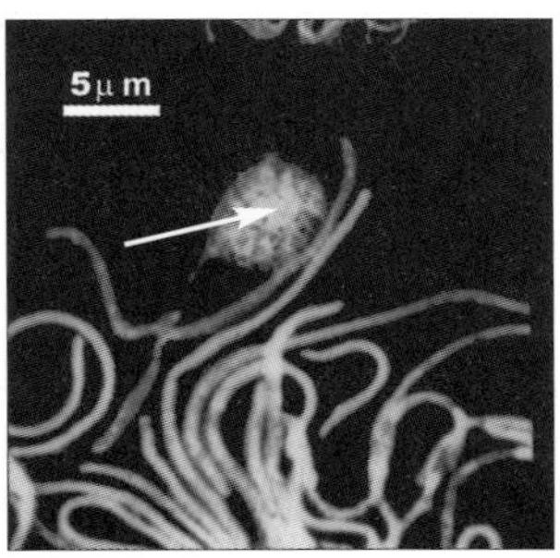

Fig. 1.2 These are impression preparations of *Spirillum serpens* showing stages in its life-cycle.

a) A young colony - 2-3 days old - that represents a so-called smooth colony of the bacteria, which have the full quota of cell-wall components, and on division the bacteria separate completely from each other.
b) An older colony referred to as rough consisting of bacteria that have lost some cell-wall components and which, on division, do not separate completely from one another and form filaments.
c) An older colony in which an early cyst form is present (arrow).
d) In this older colony a more advanced cyst-form is present (arrow). Bar = 5µm

More detail is apparent in these electron-microscope preparations of the same strain of the *Spirillum* shown on the previous page. These were grown upon collodion membranes on nutrient agar and these were captured on grids, which were then gold/palladium shadowed in order to increase the contrast and to give some impression of height. In fact the 'shadows' show up as white.

Fig. 1.3 Electron-microscopy of *S.serpens* Demonstrating its Life-cycle

a) b) c) d)

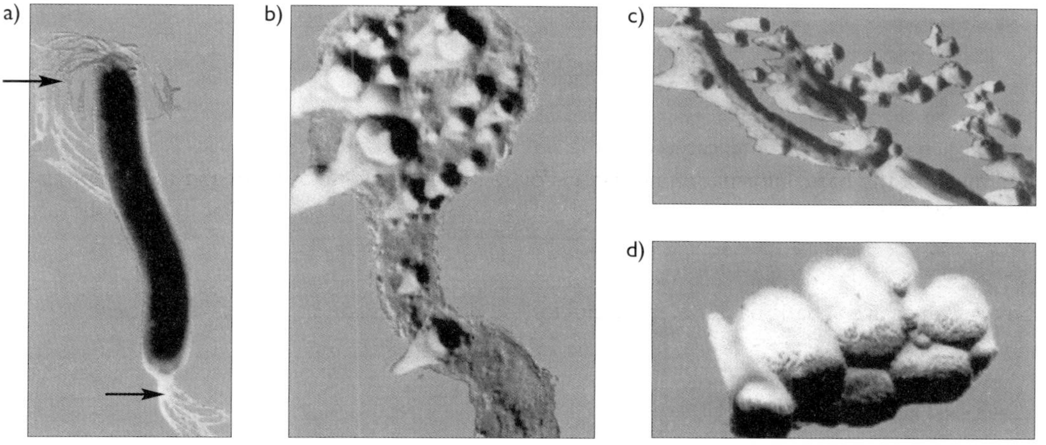

Fig 1.3a represents a single spirillum, from a smooth colony in which the cell-wall components are intact. Polar flagella are also in evidence (arrows).

b) This is an advanced cyst equivalent to the one shown in Fig. 1.2d (above) The increased resolution provided by the electron-microscope enables the examination of the cyst contents. These consist of granules of varying sizes some of which are capable of reproduction.

c) This shows the beginning of the reversion on the part of the granular forms to new whole parent forms of spirilla.

d) A small colony resulting from the division of an individual granule.

Originally the granular forms were called gonidia since some, at least, become motile but later such forms became known as L-forms. This term was coined with the discovery of tiny colonies in cultures of an unusually pleomorphic bacterium - *Streptobacillus moniliformis*, the causative agent of rat-bite fever - resembling mycoplasmas (Chapter Two), which in the long run proved to be part of the bacterial life-cycle. Klieneberger (1935) who made this discovery named them L-forms after the Lister Institute where she was then working, and this name is still in use today to describe various sub-cellular bacterial elements.

However, some authors prefer the term cell-wall-deficient (CWD) forms and this is more appropriate since the process of cell wall loss tends to be relative rather than absolute. We found proof of the usefulness of this nomenclature, in our laboratory, when we made electron sections of *Yersinia enterocolitica* in the course of our studies on Crohn's Disease. This technique revealed contents that according to Luc Montagnier (1992) resemble retroviruses.
(Pease 1979)

During these studies we used two further more simple techniques for the examination of these forms that enabled the size-range to be determined, one was dark-ground microscopy and the other was Scanning Electron-microscopy (SEM) (Pease 1981).

Fig. 1.4 Demonstration CWD forms of *Yersinia enterocolitica* by Various Techniques

a)

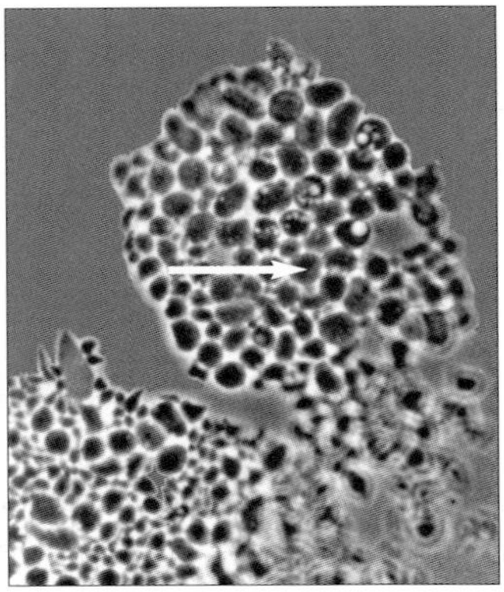

a) Dark-ground preparation of a typical small colony of *Y. enterocolitica* that occurred spontaneously during standard laboratory procedures. It is clear that the elements range in size - the larger ones are referred to as 'Large Bodies' (arrow)

b)

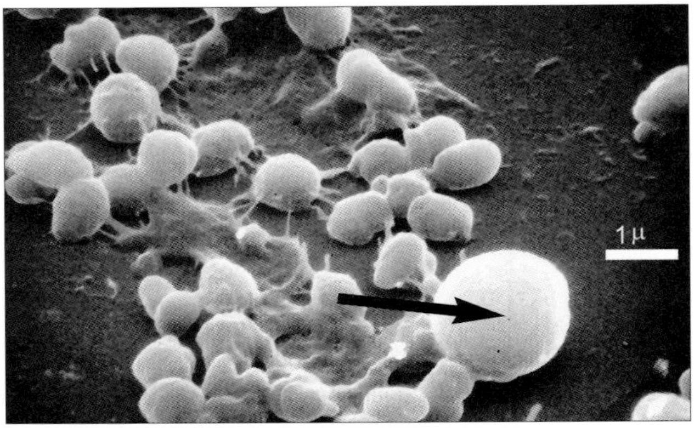

b) SEM preparation made from the sort of colony as a) showing exactly the same elements. The arrow indicates a 'Large Body' as visualised by SEM. In electron-sections viewed by transmission electron-microscopy much smaller elements resembling viruses were seen.

c)

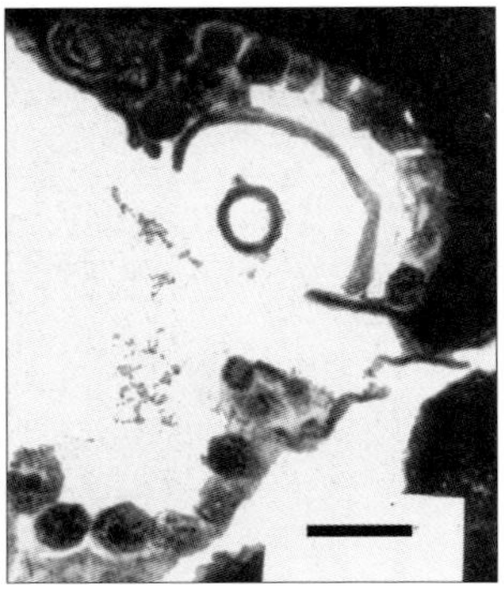

c) An electron-section of a 'Large Body' revealing tiny virus-like particles that resemble retroviruses (Montagnier 1992). It is apparent that retrovirologists were not aware of the need to exclude such sub-bacterial elements from their investigation into the cause of AIDS, some four years after the publication of the paper describing this phenomenon. This is analysed in greater detail in Chapter Eight where it is suggested that retroviruses are in fact sub-cellular elements of bacteria.

Bar = 300 nm.

Generally speaking, CWD forms tend to be more nutritionally exacting than their parents, especially when the cell-wall loss is complete, but resemble their parent bacteria, except in the antigenic and pathogenic (in conventional infections) properties that depend on cell-wall components and flagella. They sometimes occur spontaneously in culture, and can be induced in most bacteria when grown in the presence of inhibitory agents, notably antibiotics that interfere with bacterial cell-wall formation. However, whether they are spontaneous or induced, not all bacterial L-form colonies have the classical mycoplasma colonial morphology (Chapter Two), although many do.

PARASITES AND GENETICS OF BACTERIA

A further, and in the present context, crucial, characteristic that bacteria share with other biological groups is that they can be parasitized by agents unrelated to themselves and effectively are subject to epidemics as are human beings. The two main infective agents are plasmids (extra-chromosomal DNA) and bacterial viruses (bacteriophages).

Both types cause an NGE effect at the microbial level, in as much as each involves the transfer of genetic material from one organism to another, resulting in a permanent heritable change in the characteristics of the recipient. A demonstration of a plasmid epidemic in action was provided during our experiments on *Pseudomonas maltophilia* (Pease *et al* 1989), another organism suspected at one time of having a causative role in Crohn's disease.

The CWD/ L-forms were successfully induced by growing the bacteria on medium containing carbenicillin and polyvinyl pyrrolidone but maintenance in the L-form stage became extremely difficult because reversion rates became very rapid and the revertant bacteria became increasingly resistant to the carbenicillin. On electron-microscopic investigation it became clear that the resistance to carbenicillin was a result of the transfer of plasmid DNA capable of conferring this property of resistance on the recipient bacteria. This is a form of sexuality in bacteria.

Fig. 1.5 Sexuality in Bacteria

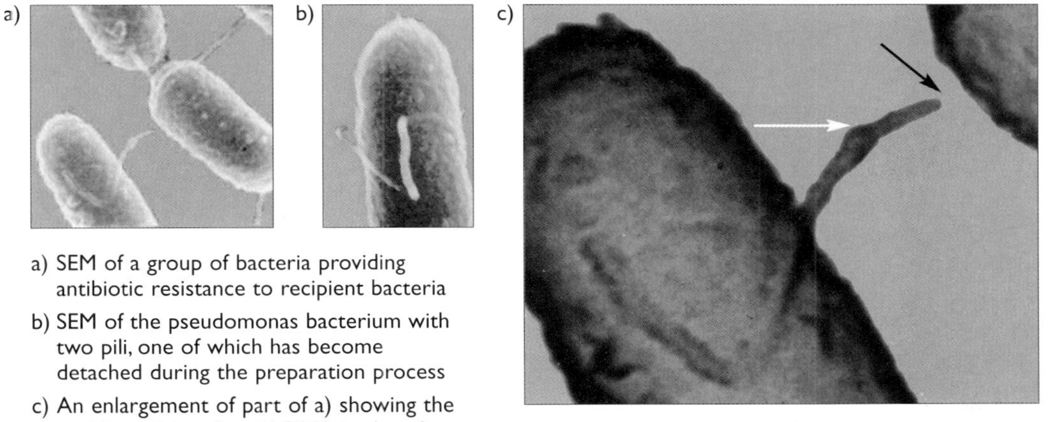

a) SEM of a group of bacteria providing antibiotic resistance to recipient bacteria
b) SEM of the pseudomonas bacterium with two pili, one of which has become detached during the preparation process
c) An enlargement of part of a) showing the position of the plasmid DNA in the pilus (white arrow) and the point at which the process was interrupted (black arrow)

Thus the bacteria are vectors (carriers) of the genetic infective elements, and understanding this bacterial function is vital to the understanding of the NGE concept of human disease.

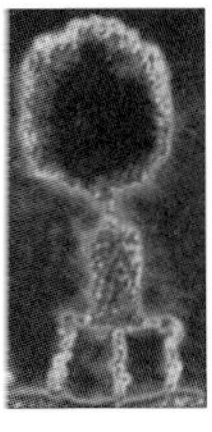

An understanding of the nature of some aspects of bacteriophage (commonly referred to as phage), which is a virus that attacks bacteria, is also important in the understanding of foreign DNA colonisation of a host nucleus. Phage particles consist of a relatively large head and a short tail, by which they become attached to the bacterium (left). In the full cycle of infection, *i.e.* when the phage is virulent, phage DNA enters the bacterium leaving the protein sheath outside, and replicates at the expense of the bacterium, which also produces the protein sheathing in proportion; complete new virus particles are formed and released by lysis (bursting) of the bacterium.

However, and more important in the present context, is the condition known as temperate or prophage, in which phage DNA can enter the host cell and replicate in rhythm with the host DNA so that the two become effectively part of the same genetic system (Fig.1.6). Some such cryptically infected bacteria are known as lysogenic because they may infect related strains with virulent phage or may be stimulated, *e.g.* by ultra violet light, to produce it themselves.

Completely latent phage DNA may confer new properties on the host cells, *e.g.* toxigenicity in *Corynebacterium diphtheriae*. Phage DNA can also act as a vehicle in the transfer of a characteristic from one bacterium to another.

Of especial interest is the case of those temperate phages which, because they have become genetically defective, are unable to revert to the virulent condition and can exist only in association with the host nucleus. In this situation the foreign phage DNA is able to replicate and confer on the host cell the ability to synthesise a varied range of virus sheath antigens (Jacob and Wollman 1961).

POSSIBLE RELATION OF BACTERIAL PARASITES TO HUMAN IMMUNOPATHOLOGIES AND MALIGNANCIES

I have previously maintained (Pease 1965), bearing in mind that these genetic exchanges are commonplace in bacteria, and that the fundamental genetic mechanisms of all cells are alike, that they are quite certain to be found in other forms of life. Furthermore that such foreign DNA colonisations brought about by means of microbial vectors could have disease-causing potential.

At that time I was referring to diseases of immune pathology, the so-called autoimmune diseases, but today it seems reasonable to investigate the possibility that some human malignant diseases can be similarly mediated, especially in view of the fact that the first such foreign DNA colonisation agents, described some years later, proved to be cancer-causing ones.

Plant cancer was found to be caused by a plasmid carried in a bacterium *i.e. Agrobacterium tumefaciens* (Chapter Three) and several avian and mammalian cancers have proved to be caused by foreign DNA carried by retroviruses (Chapter Six). These examples demonstrate yet another biological group characteristic possessed by bacteria, namely the ability to carry agents, unrelated to them and capable of causing disease in other creatures, such as the mosquito carriers of *Plasmodium vivax*, the causative agent of malaria.

The following pages describe how these examples of NGE have been exploited in the laboratory, where it has been shown that DNA's of diverse origins can be incorporated into mammalian cell nuclei including human ones. These experiments are done under very carefully controlled conditions and are directed towards 'good' causes, *e.g.* gene therapy, and are discussed in Chapter Five.

It is the philosophy behind this book that the corresponding uncontrolled NGE without restraints, left to itself, could be the cause of those diseases where infective agents seem to be involved but in a manner well outside the current concepts of bacterial and viral infections.

Fig. 1.6 Infection of Bacteria by Bacteriophage in Both Virulent and Lysogenic Stages

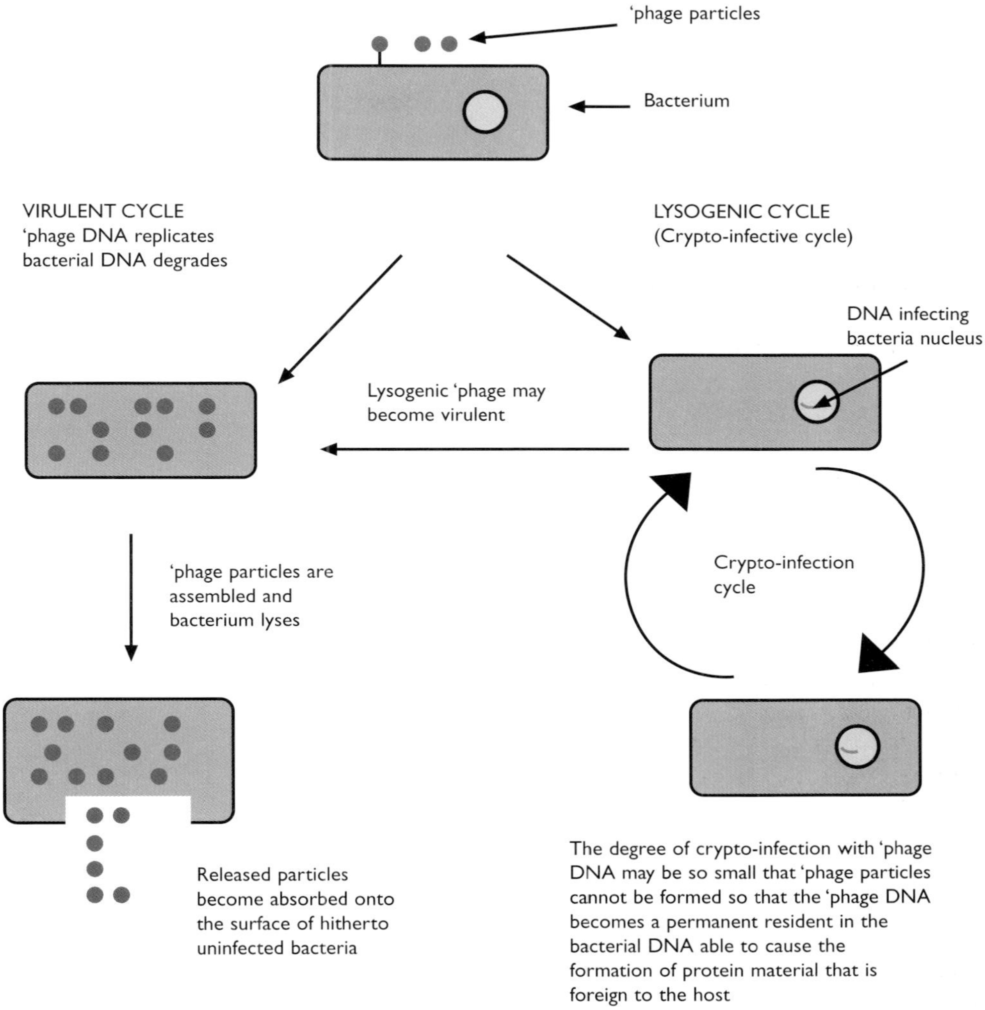

SUMMARY

In this chapter the nature of bacteria as living creatures in their own right rather than being laboratory or classical clinical agents is discussed. Their cytology and more particularly their life-cycles are described, as well as their propensity to be parasitized by DNA from alien sources. Their role as vectors in causing plant cancer is mentioned and also, by analogy, their potential as a cause of disease in humans.

REFERENCES

Beijerinck, W. M. (1925) As quoted by Heimbeck, L. S. (1963) A visit to the laboratory of Beijerinck in December 1925.
Phytopathology 53: 862

Bisset, K. A, (1952) Complete and Reduced Life Cycles in *Rhizobium*
J. gen. Microbiol. 7 233-242

Bisset, KA (1970) The Cytology and Life History of Bacteria.
E and S Livingstone - Edinburgh and London

Hadley, P. (1931) The filterable forms of bacteria. 1. A filterable stage in the life history of the Shiga dysentery bacillus
J infect. Dis 48 1

Jacob, F. and Wollman, E. L. (1961) Sexuality and Genetics of Bacteria
London and New York: Academic Press

Klieneberger, E. (1935) The natural occurrence of pleuropneumonia-like organisms in apparent symbiosis with *Streptobacillus moniliformis* and other bacteria
J. Path. Bact. 40 93-105

Pease, Phyllis. (1956) The Gonidial Stages in *Spirillum* spp. and *Vibrio* spp.
J. Medical Microbiol. 14 672-675

Pease, P. E. (1965) L-Forms, Episomes and Autoimmune Disease,
E. & S Livingstone Ltd, Edinburgh and London

Pease, Phyllis. (1979) Observations on L-forms of *Yersinia enterocolitica.*
J. Med. Microbiol. 12 337-346

Pease. Phyllis. (1981) Scanning electron microscopy of L-forms of *Yersinia enterocolitica*
Microbios 31 17-23

Pease, P.E., Lawson. J.W., Bartlett, L.K. *et al* (1989) Observations on cell-wall deficient forms of *Pseudomonas maltophilia*
Microbios. 57 21-26

Smith, D.C. (1979). From extracellular to intracellular, the establishment of a symbiosis
Proc R. Soc Lond. 204 115-130

Note added in proof

NANOBACTERIA

In the next Chapter I have written at some length about the (now) well-known phenomenon of contamination of culture media particularly tissue cultures and of animal, including human, bloods with mycoplasmas.

Currently evidence has accumulated that putative CWD bacteria occur in similar habitats and are therefore also likely to cause serious problems of interpretation if undetected.

The naming of these agents as nanobacteria giving the false impression that they constitute a novel type of microorganism has been most unfortunate.Small filterable bacteria have been recognised since the end of the 19th century and measurements in nanometres of these has been commonplace in the last century as I have described in this Chapter.

The nanobacteria-like structures associated with precipitation of calcium carbonate were first described by geologists in natural hotspring deposits in Italy - the name nanoparticles being so-named because of their small size (0.03-0.3mm i.e. 30-300nm - see Figs.1.4c and 2.2e.) Similar structures have apparently been found in human blood, urine, renal cyst fluid and kidney stones and demonstrated by electron-microscopy in ovarian cancer specimens (see Miller et al 2004 for references).

Clearly these structures are worthy of further investigation. Several questions need to be resolved e.g.if the particles, which appear to be able to reproduce, are bacterial, are they related to the bacteria discussed in this book?; do they have a role in disease causation?; do they have deficient cell-walls? does filtration of material containing the particles hold back larger bacterial forms capable of reproduction?.

My own observations on the life-cycle Yersinia enterocolitica strongly suggest that the structures in the calcified human arteries and cardiac valves described by Miller et al are indeed CWD bacterial forms.These observations will be the subject of another publication.

Miller,V.M., Rodgers, G., Charlesworth, Jon A.et al (2004) Evidence of nanobacterial-like structures in calcified human arteries and cardiac valves
Am.J. Heart Circ Physiol 287 1115-1124

Wainwright, M. (1999) Nanobacteria and the associated 'elementary bodies' in human disease and cancer
Microbiology 145 2623-26

CHAPTER TWO

THE MYCOPLASMAS

'Pease, your mycoplasma laboratory will be situated as far away from the virological ones (Smallpox and Herpes) as possible and neither you, nor any of your staff, will be allowed in these laboratories at any time.'

(P Wildy to author 1964)

INTRODUCTION	24
MORPHOLOGY OF MYCOPLASMAS	26
MYCOPLASMA CONTAMINATION OF TISSUE AND OTHER CULTURE MEDIA	28
SOURCES OF MYCOPLASMA CONTAMINATION	29
MYCOPLASMAS AS CONTAMINANTS IN AIDS RESEARCH	29
THE 'PERMISSIVE' H9 CELL-LINE	31
THE ACQUISITION OF CELLULAR PERMISSIVENESS FOR MYCOPLASMA GROWTH	32
ELECTRON-MICROSCOPY OF MYCOPLASMA AND HIV CO-INFECTION	33
MYCOPLASMAS FROM AIDS PATIENTS	34
HAEMOPLASMAS	35
SUMMARY	35

INTRODUCTION

Mycoplasmas are a fascinating group of cell-wall-less bacteria, which have over many years been the cause of several disappointments in the search for the causes of human diseases. They have been recognised for over a hundred years, the first recorded one being the causative agent of contagious pneumonia of cattle in 1898, but it was not until the discovery of a type that causes primary atypical pneumonia (PAP) in humans (*Mycoplasma pneumoniae*) by Chanock *et al* in 1962 that any serious attention was paid to them by the medical research community. In both of these cases the initial interpretation was that the causative agents were viruses, since they were able to pass through filters designed to hold back bacteria, and it was only when attempts were made to grow them on serum or other body-fluid enriched solid medium that it was understood that they were in fact what is now known as mycoplasmas. They grew as tiny and delicate colonies often called 'fried-egg like', resembling those in Fig.2.1a.

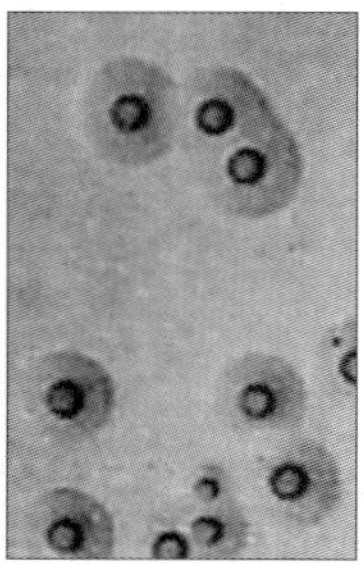
Fig. 2.1a

Whilst they resemble the sub-cellular forms of walled bacteria discussed in the last chapter, mycoplasmas do not have a walled stage and their connection with classic bacteria goes back into antiquity, their origins appearing to be in the gram positive bacteria (Neimark 1996).

However, in the present context this is not the main concern since both types of organism have phases in which they are capable of passing through bacterial filters, and the lack of rigid cell wall material causes their elements to be fragile and flexible so that they can easily escape detection by the untutored research worker. This is particularly likely to happen in research in which tissue cultures are employed, a fact widely appreciated in the sixties after the first report of the phenomenon by Robinson *et al* in 1956. After this classic report it was realised, with considerable dismay, by the then current virological research establishment including senior investigators in our laboratory that a considerable amount of virus research needed to be reappraised. The reason for this was that various characteristics, especially cytopathogenicity, which had been attributed to viruses, were in fact due to the hitherto undetected mycoplasma contamination.

Unfortunately, this information has been ignored by most AIDS research workers, and ever since the realisation that mycoplasmas have sometimes been closely associated with AIDS, their precise role in the disorder has remained problematical. Indeed, such has been the state of affairs in AIDS research that Montagnier and Blanchard (1993) when discussing the finding that neurotoxic properties initially attributed to HIV could not be reproduced in mycoplasma free conditions, wrote 'This case clearly shows that the testing of cell cultures and virus stock for mycoplasmal contamination is not a current practice in AIDS research'. This was ten years after the first recognition of the epidemic, and clearly covers the time during which the most vital early steps of isolation and identification of HIV took place. This flaw in AIDS research has never been addressed seriously by that research community and the significance of this is discussed below.

Mycoplasma contamination of viral growth media was at the basis of many of the disappointments in the search for a mycoplasma as the possible cause of human rheumatoid arthritis (RA) for instance - an idea stimulated by the discovery of *M.pneumoniae* as a human pathogen and by the fact that various mycoplasmas were known to attack the joints of sheep and goats (*Mycoplasma agalactiae*) and of laboratory animals, particularly mice. In fact, mycoplasmas are effectively as common a hazard as that presented by classic bacteria and this is exacerbated by their less obvious presence and their resistance to the normal antibiotic 'umbrellas' of streptomycin and penicillin that were common at the time.

This approach to the search for the aetiology of RA was brought to a halt when it became apparent that many of the isolates came from the constituents of the culture media - in some cases tissue cultures - and were simply contaminants. Two publications in 1974 (Stewart *et al* and Taylor-Robinson) made this explanation the most plausible although I would add the rider that mycoplasmas can occasionally be isolated from synovial fluid when all the controls are in place. I have done this myself but have regarded these observations as simply reinforcing the now accepted concept of the virtual ubiquity of mycoplasmas. Isolates from malignant tissues likewise came to be recognised as contaminants.

When the phenomenon was rediscovered by the Montagnier group, the interpretation was that although a contaminant in HIV cultures, the mycoplasmas had fortuitously provided a clue to the identity of the elusive co-factor (Chapter Eight) required for the progression from infection with HIV to advanced AIDS.

As a result of this unconventional interpretation - the customary procedure with contaminating bacteria is to discard the cultures and start again - research into the possible role of mycoplasmas in human disease has been revived to some extent and they have been implicated in such diverse conditions as the Gulf War syndrome, Chronic Fatigue syndrome and Crohn's disease. Interest has also been renewed in their possible role in RA and malignant disease (Baseman and Tully 1997). However it has become apparent that mycoplasmas can be found in most environments observers feel worth investigating.

In addition to medical research workers interested in investigating mycoplasmas as causes of diseases other than PAP, the microorganisms have also been recognised as the cause of plant diseases. As is so often the case in research, the first reports of these forms of bacteria as causative agents of plant diseases were ignored, and some thirty years later the phenomenon was re-discovered. This was after the renewal of interest in them as potential human pathogens and illustrates the unfortunate artificial divide that existed in most of the twentieth century between agricultural and medical bacteriology. This artificial division is discussed further in Chapter Seven with respect to the lessons to be learnt from a comparative study of plant and human cancers and the bacteria associated with them.

The attention of chemists, biochemists and molecular biologists was also drawn to the mycoplasmas largely on account of their being the smallest organisms capable of independent life. As a result, reports on mycoplasmas have been widely published in journals concerned with nucleic acid research.

Information about these organisms is now so widespread in the scientific literature and so voluminous that there is a case for reviews of reviews. Razin *et al* (1998) covered molecular biological and pathogenicity aspects and listed several other reviews covering others, and the one by Baseman and Tully (1997) mentioned above is an interesting easily readable one covering historical aspects as well as more recent information about research trends.

In the present context my aim is simply to indicate the ways in which mycoplasmas can infiltrate experiments and give rise to erroneous results that have led to serious misconceptions in AIDS research in particular. Electron-microscopy, the *sine qua non* of virus investigation, has never been satisfactorily carried out in the case of retroviruses. In some published electron-micrographs it is clear that mycoplasmas are present in supposedly pure cultures of the retroviruses, and it seems very probable that the smaller mycoplasma particles have been mistaken for retroviruses.

Since the discovery of reverse transcriptase (RT) and with it the birth of retrovirology (Chapter Five), surrogate biochemical markers, especially the presence of RT, have replaced rather than complemented the essential first class electron-microscopic scrutiny of preparations of viruses for the determination of their presence and purity, and this has led to a great deal of slipshod work.

In fact, the poor controls for contaminating mycoplasmas, combined with the fact that the standard methods for the isolation of retroviruses do not remove cellular debris (Chapters Five, Eight and Nine), have cast doubts in the eyes of some investigators on the true nature of retroviruses.

The emphasis in this chapter is on the visual appearance of mycoplasmas and the viruses with which they have been confused, especially the human retroviruses.

MORPHOLOGY OF MYCOPLASMAS

As is the case when handling the sub-cellular elements of walled bacteria, gentle handling is necessary to get a good indication of their true morphology. However, because some elements/particles are so small - 0.1 µm or even less, electron-microscopy, which involves quite harsh treatment, is needed to visualise these elements.

Much time and effort has been spent over the years in trying to work out the life-cycles of mycoplasmas, but all that is needed in the present context is to understand something about the morphology of these organisms so that they may be recognised in blood and tissues. Also it is necessary to see in some detail how they might be confused with retrovirus particles.

The following electron-micrographs show the characteristics of mycoplasmas as demonstrated by different techniques. Differences in the preparations, such as whether the starting material consisted of mycoplasmas grown in fluid or on solid agar, and whether sectioned or not show up different aspects of mycoplasma morphology. The degree of pleomorphism exhibited by these organisms is so great - the elements of which range in size from less than 100 nm to greater than 5 µm, that they can be confused with virus particles at one extreme and blood cells at the other.

The technique used to demonstrate the mycoplasma elements shown in Fig.2.2a (which represent whole elements *i.e.* non-sectioned) is useful in demonstrating such elements on the surface of human erythrocytes (Chapter Three).

Figs. 2.2a to 2.2e Morphology of Mycoplasmas

Fig. 2.2a

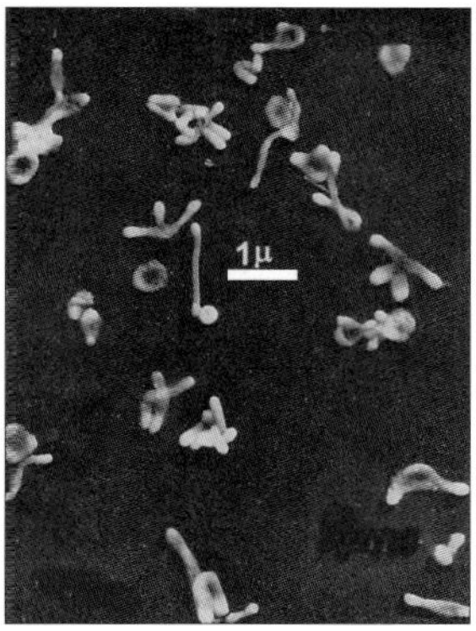

This is an electron-micrograph of a mycoplasma adapted from one produced by Emmy Klieneberger-Nobel (1956). The preparation was made from a broth culture and shows characteristic ring forms and filaments.

Fig. 2.2.b

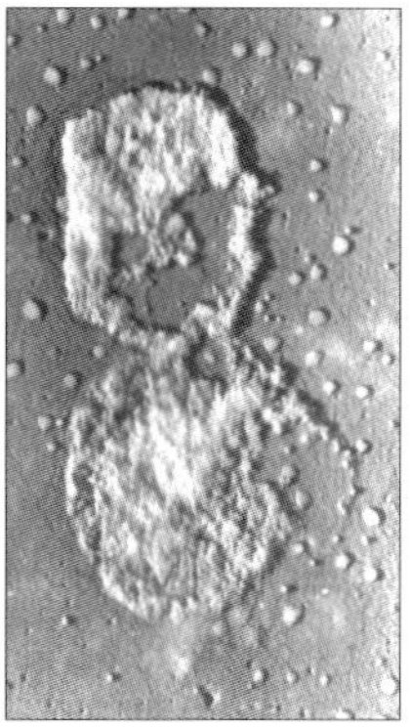

This is an electron-micrograph produced in our laboratory of a mycoplasma isolated from the lung of a stillborn child. It is an impression preparation made from a culture growing on solid medium. The two large particles are about 2-3μm in diameter, whilst the small ones fall within the range of retrovirus sizes.

Fig. 2.2c

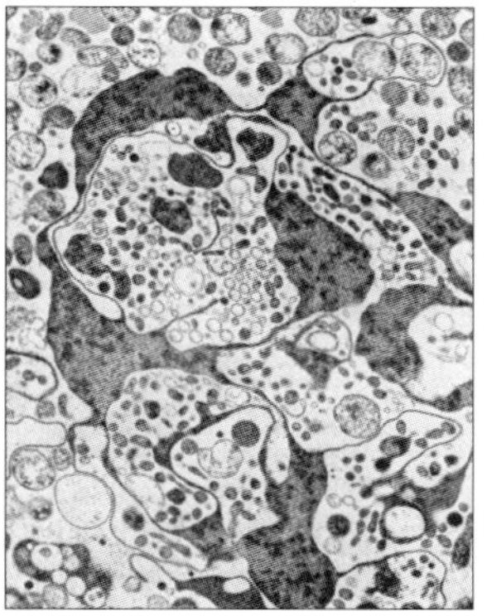

This is a section of a mycoplasma isolated from a human and grown in fluid medium. The 'Large Body' (LB) here takes up most of the electron-micrograph and it contains particles of varying sizes. There are also numerous particles outside it. The LB could easily be mistaken for a blood cell and the smaller ones for retroviruses. (After Anderson 1969).

Fig. 2.2d

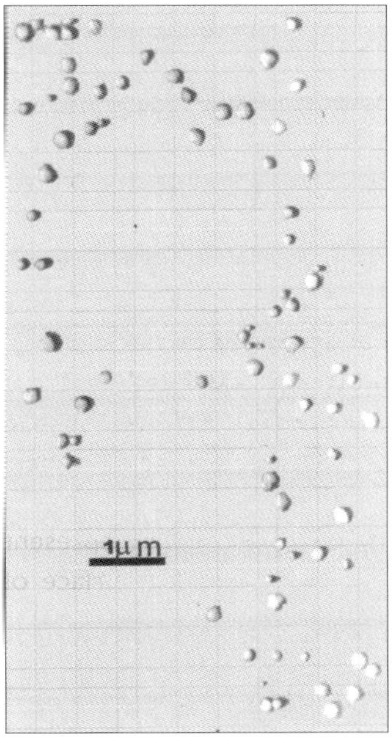

Fig. 2.2d is derived from Fig. 2.2b and shows the effect of filtration as used in the preparation of so-called retrovirus isolation (Chapter Eight). Filtration effectively removes most of the larger elements thus giving a false impression.

Fig. 2.2e

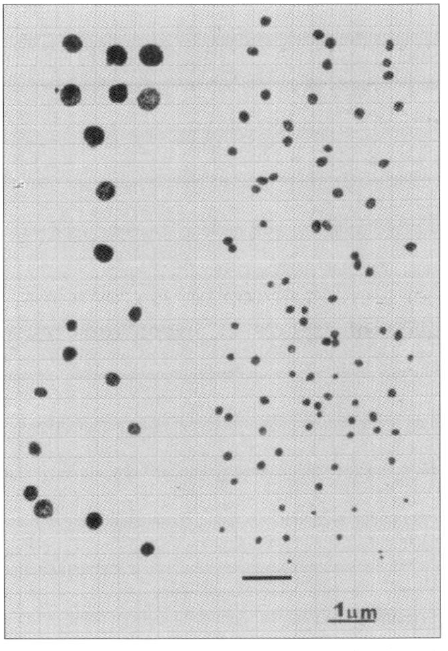

Fig. 2.2e shows TEM sections of particles of *mycoplasma hominis* grown in fluid medium derived from 2.2c.

An analysis of the particle sizes shown in Fig. 2.2e gives an idea of the size range of the smaller mycoplasma particles and illustrates how some could easily be mistaken for retroviruses. Most particles are unlikely to be viable but some 'minimal reproductive units' (mrus) exist. The smallest particles are clearly able to pass through the filters used for the isolation of retroviruses, leaving behind the larger elements and giving the wrong impression.

The possibility that other forms of cell-wall less bacteria have been confused with retroviruses is discussed in Chapters Five and Eight.

MYCOPLASMA CONTAMINATION OF TISSUE AND OTHER CULTURE MEDIA

Robinson *et al* (1956) made the discovery that mycoplasma contamination is widespread during their investigations into the effects of human and animal mycoplasmas on the types of tissue cultures available in their laboratory. They found that the uninoculated control cultures were already supporting the growth of contaminating mycoplasmas and suspected, almost certainly correctly, that the contamination arose from some common constituent of the culture media. They foresaw the problems that the undetected presence of mycoplasmas could cause, such as the invalidating or confusing of results in virological experiments, and suggested the use of routine testing of cultures and media for mycoplasmas. They also recommended the incorporation of 'a suitable level of one of the antibiotics of the tetracycline series' as an aid to the prevention of mycoplasma contamination. In fact, the main points concerning the detection and control of the mycoplasma problem were all clearly stated in this relatively short communication.

The contamination of tissue cultures with mycoplasmas may cause cytopathogenic effects and influence cell-growth. The cells may be almost entirely unaffected, or only slightly as in the case of cells investigated by the Robinson group, or there may be widespread killing of cells. The growth rate of the cells may also be retarded (see below). One of the earliest studies reporting severe cell damage with accompanying acidity caused by mycoplasma contaminating and effectively destroying tissue culture cells was done by Butler and Leach (1964). Of considerable interest is that no appreciable acidity or cytopathogenicity was observed when the medium was replaced at regular three to four day intervals. The reason for the interest being that a similar tactic was adopted by Hoxie *et al* (1985) in the prolonged culturing of normal lymphocytes in the presence of HIV (referred to as ARV in the paper) and their success in this endeavour may have been due likewise to the suppression of mycoplasmas.

A further area of potential confusion involving mycoplasma contamination that merits some discussion is that some mycoplasmas cause chromosome changes that could in certain circumstances be wrongly attributed. Paton *et al* (1965) observed chromosome aberrations in a human diploid cell line (strain WI-38) which normally retained a diploid complement of chromosomes for up to some forty passages. The aberrations observed were; high polyploidy and break frequencies and some cells with fragmented chromosomes and there was a concomitant slowing down of cell growth. The cultures were found to contain a mycoplasma, and subsequent experiments showed that mycoplasmas could indeed change cell chromosomes. Since viruses in cell cultures as well as in blood cultures can induce chromosome damage similar to that described, the authors felt the need to reiterate the need for caution in interpreting experimental results without adequately testing for the presence of mycoplasmas.

SOURCES OF MYCOPLASMA CONTAMINATION

It is important to know the possible sources of contamination in order to install an efficient mycoplasma testing facility. It is necessary to test the following areas, bearing in mind that several of the substances used in tissue culture are unsuitable for autoclaving, and that the standard filtration techniques used for the 'sterilisation' of body fluids will not hold back the smaller mycoplasma and other cell-wall defective elements.

a) It is essential to test the cell culture containing the virus of interest for contamination before using it. This applies whatever the source, be it from another research laboratory, or a National Type collection of cell-lines

b) It is essential to test the new tissue or fluid from which the line originates for mycoplasmas at the stage of the founding of a cell-line. Cell-lines derived from tumour tissues fluids are particularly likely to contain mycoplasmas from the original source, hence the initial excitement at the possibility of them being the cause of some cancers.

c) It is vitally important to test all fluids used in the process of tissue culture for contamination. This is especially true for serum from a wide variety of animals as well as humans.

d) Laboratory workers may be a source of contamination, but this is largely avoidable by the application of good laboratory practice.

e) It is necessary to avoid contamination between cell-lines. This is practicable only if cell-lines and the personnel working with them are confined to separate rooms.

In summary, the only safe method for avoiding the potential devastation that can be wrought by mycoplasma contamination in a virological or other relevant laboratory is the installation of a mandatory screening facility (Wildy 1964).

MYCOPLASMAS AS CONTAMINANTS IN AIDS RESEARCH

These crucial screening procedures were not carried out in the early stages of AIDS research or even as late as 1993 (Montagnier and Blanchard). Thus for ten years at least, and judging by a study of the literature, probably up to the time of writing, HIV culture work has not always been properly controlled. This problem arises mostly in tissue cell lines but it can occur in fresh lymphocyte cultures as well, and also in cord lymphocytes where infection from mother to child may take place. The implications of this situation, which do not seem to have been understood by the AIDS research community, are discussed further in Chapter Eight.
The Montagnier group (LeMaître *et al* 1990) encountered (re-discovered) mycoplasma

contamination of tissue cell-lines in studies on various compounds in a search for drugs less toxic than AZT for the treatment of AIDS. These experiments showed that tetracycline treatment of the CEM cells blocked the growth of contaminating mycoplasmas and allowed the tissue cells to grow without damage. In fact this paper demonstrates simply, elegantly and clearly, a vital piece of information, *i.e.* that *in vitro* HIV is not cytopathogenic.

The work was published in a little known French publication and presumably escaped the attention of many AIDS investigators. It attracted much more interest on the part of the mycoplasma research workers.

Fig. 2.3 The Viability of CEM cells in the Presence and Absence of Tetracyclines (After Le Maître et *al*)

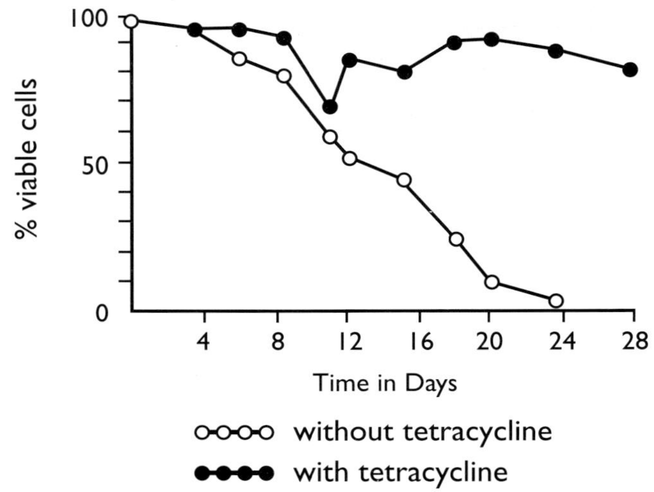

This graph shows clearly that the cell-killing properties attributed to HIV on the cell culture (known as CEM - a T-cell line derived from the leukaemic cells of a child with acute lymphoid leukaemia - Chapter Seven) were due to the unrecognised mycoplasma contaminant of the cell-line. In the presence of tetracycline analogues, which inactivate mycoplasmas the cells were healthy - without these the cells died rapidly.

Fig. 2.4 The Cytopathogenic Effects (CPE) of Mycoplasma

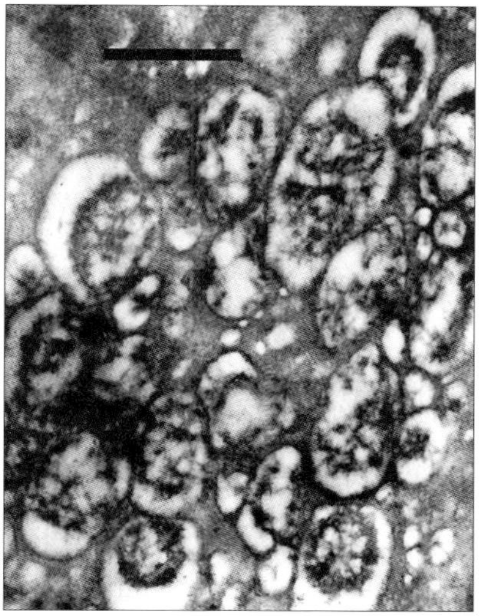

The mycoplasma figured here was isolated from the lung of a stillborn child (Fig. 2.2b). The cytopathogenic effect (CPE) was very obvious and killed most of the cells. The presence of tetracycline analogues in the tissue cells (Hep2-cell-line) could prevent the CPE since it deactivates mycoplasma activity.

Instead of this sounding a note of caution with respect to the pathogenicity of HIV, however, as it would have done thirty years before, the discovery by the Montagnier group was interpreted as the unearthing of the co-factor that seemed to be needed to explain the progression from HIV infection to the onset of advanced AIDS.

The same group (Le Maitre *et al* 1992) later confirmed that the cytopathogenic effects in both lymphoblastoid cells (CEM) and promonocytic cells (U937) of HIV-1 occurred only in the presence of mycoplasma contamination. Moreover, HIV-1 infection of U937 after experimental inoculation with a human isolate of *M.fermentans*, isolated from an HIV sero-positive patient (AOU) 'led to pronounced cell killing'. The explanation advanced by Montagnier and his collaborators for this phenomenon was that the contaminating mycoplasma assisted HIV in its cytopathogenicity and was a necessary co-factor for the CPE.

Montagnier and Blanchard (1993) pursued this idea in a review article, in which they advanced the hypothesis that the origin of the AIDS epidemic lay in the meeting of two infective agents: HIV that issued from African countries and mycoplasmas from elsewhere. They suggested that this as a possible explanation for the problem that has dogged AIDS research from the time of the discovery of HIV *i.e.* the variability of the time course that elapses between the time of presumed infection with HIV and the onset of clinical AIDS (Chapters Eight and Nine).

THE 'PERMISSIVE' H9 CELL-LINE

The H9 cell-line is the most well known one in AIDS research. It was developed by the Gallo group - famous for being the co-discoverers of HIV (Chapter Eight) - for the specific purpose of allowing (permitting) the growth of this allegedly cell-killing agent. This was urgently needed to study the characteristics of the putative virus and in the long run to develop a vaccine to prevent AIDS spreading throughout the world.

The classic explanation - still accepted (Moore 2002) - provided in the famous 1984 papers by the Gallo group, effectively announcing the discovery of the causative agent of AIDS, was that H9 and some other cell-lines had become resistant to the putative HIV. This is clearly a misinterpretation. The true explanation, discussed further in Chapter Eight, is clearly that the cells became resistant to the contaminating mycoplasma and not to the non-cytopathogenic HIV.

This explanation is supported by the observation of critical importance reported in the Le Maitre *et al* paper is that 'infection of H9 cells with HIV did not produce CPE and the experimental contamination with *M.fermentans* did not change this feature'. In other words, the H9 cells were resistant to mycoplasma infection.

This is supported visually in the Garry images of control HIV infected cells, which were sub-clones of H9 in which the mycoplasmas are growing without any noticeable effect upon the RH9 cells (Chapter Eight).

In fact, this misinterpretation has had very far reaching and unfortunate effects in the investigations on AIDS because the belief that the cells of H9 are permissive for HIV growth as opposed to being permissive for mycoplasma growth has led to the very widespread use of this particular cell-line in all sorts of research areas e.g. in much of the work on simian AIDS. Indeed it is probable that the use of H9 cells has undermined the findings in untold numbers of research projects.

THE ACQUISITION OF CELLULAR PERMISSIVENESS FOR MYCOPLASMA GROWTH

Since the occurrence of mycoplasma contamination of tissue cultures usually leads to the simple expedient of discarding the offending cell-cultures and starting experiments over again, there are very few studies on the problem of cells becoming resistant to the effects of mycoplasma cytopathogenicity. One of these studies was conducted by Fogh *et al* in 1965, who wrote that many of the morphological changes in the tissue cells such as their rounding up and their detachment from the glass provided an impression that 'could easily be mistaken for cytopathic (sic) virus effects'. Most of the study was concerned with their established FL human amnion line in which very striking effects of mycoplasma infection were observed. These results were also presented in the form of graphs (Fig, 2.5).

Cells surviving the mycoplasma infection could be sub-cultured and continued to grow at the slower rate. These cells could be maintained with infrequent transfers up to 12 months and most of the cell population remained healthy even though the mycoplasmas were present in high titres and could easily be demonstrated in the culture fluids. These surviving cells grew in tightly packed colonies and compared with uninfected populations show more variation in size. Occasional giant cells occurred, some cells were vacuolated and some were spindle shaped. These observations are consistent with the theory that the cell-line developed in the Gallo laboratory (H9) alleged to be resistant to the CPE effects of HIV was in fact a cell-line that had developed resistance to contaminating mycoplasmas.

Fig. 2.5 The Acquisition of Resistance to the Cytopathogenic Effects (CPE) of Mycoplasmas by Tissue-culture cells (After Fogh et *al*)

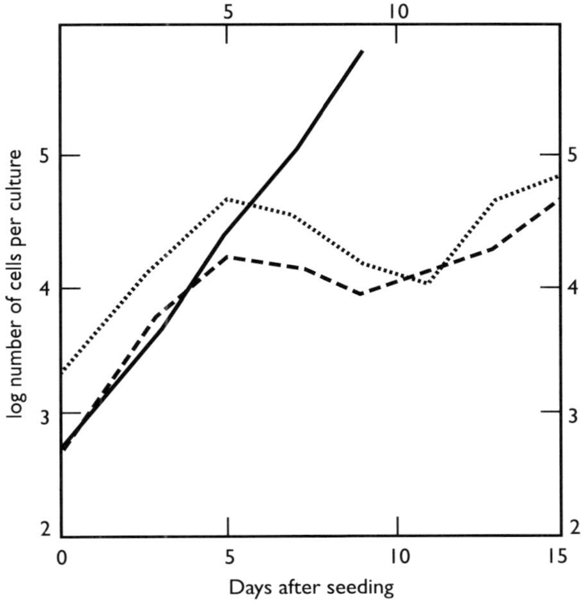

Fig 2.5 This graph illustrates the growth of FL human amnion cells both contaminated and uncontaminated with mycoplasmas. Continuous line - uncontaminated, Broken lines - contaminated. The cells were seeded at two levels (500 and 2000 cells per flask) in Bodian's medium + 20% human serum. For infection 10,000 colony forming units (CFUs) were inoculated immediately after cell-seeding. Cells were counted every second day. During the first 5 days the number of cells per culture increased to the same extent in infected and uninfected cultures apparently logarithmically. From day 5 the population of the infected cultures started to decrease for about 5 days. A further increase in cell numbers occurred after 10 days and the rate of growth in this infected population was much lower than that of the uninfected population.

The crucial point in this work in the present context is that the loss of the CPE trait enabled the mycoplasma to live freely and inconspicuously in the culture, enabling it to continue to cause confusion with co-cultivated viruses in their capacity as antigenic and biochemical agents. In this case, the mycoplasmas were easy to grow in cell-free medium and further experiments showed that even at high concentrations the cell resistance remained unaffected by their presence.

ELECTRON-MICROSCOPY OF MYCOPLASMA AND HIV CO-INFECTION

Electron-microscope studies on HIV-infected lymphocyte cultures that became contaminated with mycoplasma have provided some interesting results in this area (Phillips *et al* 1992). These studies emphasise the extremely close relationship between mycoplasmas and human retroviruses. The authors used a quantitative morpho-metric technique to analyse electron-micrographs taken of human T-cells infected both with mycoplasmas and one of two human retroviruses *i.e.* either HIV or HTLV (Chapter Five). The interest of these observations lies in the fact that the T-cells associated with the retroviruses were much more likely to be associated with mycoplasmas than those that were not. Furthermore, the two types of organism *i.e.* retrovirus and mycoplasma, were observed in the same region of the cell in ninety per cent of cases.

Fig. 2.6 Electron-sections of T-cells infected with Mycoplasmas and Retroviruses (After Phillips et *al* 1992, with permission)

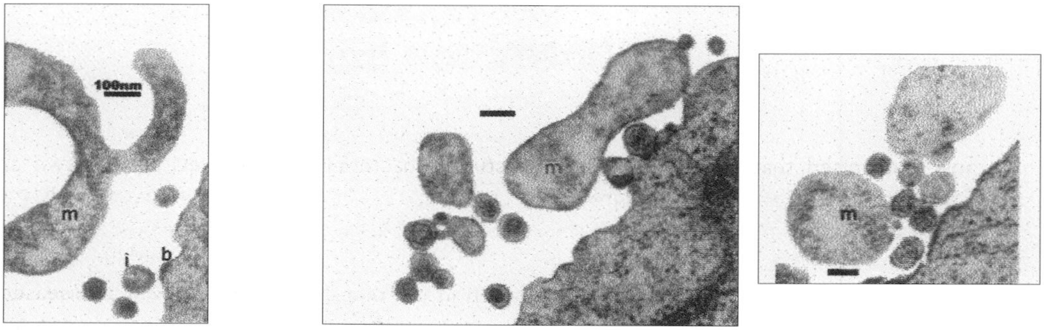

Fig. 2.6a MOLT -4 culture infected with HIV and mycoplasma (m) Budding (b) or immature (i). HIV virions in the same regions as the mycoplasmas.

Figs. 2.6b and 2.6c HTLV associated with mycoplasma on the surface of MT cells. In almost every instance when HTLV and mycoplasmas are observed together they occur at the same region of the cell periphery. Fig. 2.6c is reproduced in Chapter Eight for purposes of further comparison with the range of sizes of HIV and contaminating mycoplasmas.

These results underline still more the likelihood of confusion occurring between the two groups of organisms, not only concerning the correct attribution of cytopathogenicity but also of serological specificities (Chapter Six) and in the preparation of 'purified' virus preparations by the methods employed for retrovirus isolation and analysis, which is discussed in Chapters Five and Eight.

MYCOPLASMAS FROM AIDS PATIENTS

Another group, Lo *et al* (1989) also came across mycoplasmas in their researches into AIDS but their approach was from a different angle. They were investigating DNA extracted from a Kaposi sarcoma in a transfection experiment using the NIH 3T3 tissue line (Chapter Five) and initially believed that a transmissible agent with an outer limiting membrane and a buoyant density of 1.17-1.20 was a virus. This was later found to be a mycoplasma, first given the name *Mycoplasma incognitus* and finally identified as *Mycoplasma fermentans*. Additional studies by the group (Lo *et al* 1991) indicated that in the presence of this strain of *M.fermentans* greatly enhanced cytocidal effects occurred in HIV cultures, although syncytial formation was apparently virtually inhibited. They also discovered a truly previously unknown mycoplasma- *Mycoplasma penetrans* - first in the urine of an HIV-1 positive male homosexual patient - symptom-less except for prolonged low CD4 counts - and later from five HIV positive patients with AIDS. Ninety eight HIV-1 negative controls showed no evidence of the newly isolated mycoplasma.

These two mycoplasmas in particular, as well as several others, have been widely studied in connection with AIDS research and a great deal of information has been obtained in connection with their ability to invade cells and to activate the immune system. In general it is widely agreed that several mycoplasmas possess properties that would enable them to act as co-factors in the progression of AIDS.

However it is unlikely that they play more of a role than any other opportunist agents and are not essential to the development of AIDS.

HAEMOPLASMAS

It is now recognised that some relatively little studied bacterial species, previously known as *Haemobartonella* and *Eperithrozoon* that infect the erythrocytes of a wide range of host animals are forms of mycoplasmas that have not been hitherto cultivated in artificial medium (Rikihisa *et al* 1997, Razin *et al* 1998, Neimark *et al* 2002). Furthermore, there has been evidence available for over thirty years that similar organisms are very common in the blood of normal as well as diseased humans. These bacteria, which give rise to further concern about lack of microbiological controls in AIDS, are discussed in the next chapter.

SUMMARY

In this chapter a description, with particular emphasis on morphology of mycoplasmas is provided, and their potential as pathogens, usually secondary but occasionally primary, as a cause of atypical pneumonia for example is briefly discussed. The main emphasis, however, is on their potentially disastrous propensity to contaminate materials, especially tissue cultures used to culture viruses. Although this phenomenon was well recognised in the sixties, awareness of it in AIDS research has been almost completely lacking. The ability of cell-lines to become resistant to mycoplasmas, rendering the contaminants 'silent', is also discussed with reference to AIDS research.

REFERENCES

Anderson, D.R. (1969) Ultra-structural Studies of Mycoplasmas and the L-Phase of Bacteria in The Mycoplasmas and the L-Phase of Bacteria
North Holland Publishing Company - Amsterdam

Baseman, J.B., and Tully, J.G. (1997) Mycoplasmas: Sophisticated, Re-emerging, and Burdened by their Notoriety
Emerging Infectious Diseases 3 1-14

Brenner, C., Neyrolles, O and Blanchard, A. (1996) Mycoplasmas and HIV Infection: From Epidemiology to Their Interaction with Immune Cells
Frontiers in Bioscience 1 42-54

Butler, M. and Leach, R.H. (1964) A Mycoplasma which induces Acidity and Cytopathic Effect in Tissue Culture.
J gen. Microbiol. 34 285-294

Chanock, R.M., Hayflick, L. and Barile, M.F. (1962) Growth on artificial medium of an agent associated with atypical pneumonia and its identification as a PPLO. Proc.
Nat Acad Sci. 48 41

Chastel, C. (1995) Links and interactions between mycoplasmas and viruses: past confusions and present realities
Archives of Virology 140 811-826

Collier, L.H. (1957) Contamination of stock lines of human carcinoma cells by pleuropneumonia-like organisms
Nature 180 757-758

Fogh, E., Hahn, E. and Fogh, H. (1965) Effects of Pleuropneumonia-like Organisms on Cultured Human Cells
Experimental Cell Research 39 554-567

Hoxie, J.A., Haggarty, B.S., Rakowsky, J.L. *et al* (1985) persistent non-cytopathic infection of normal human T lymphocytes with AIDS-associated retrovirus
Science 229 1400-1402

Klienberger-Nobel E. and Cuckow, F.W. (1955) A study of organisms of the pleuropneumonia group by electron-microscopy
J gen Microbiol 12 95

Lemaitre, M., Guetard, D., Henin, Y. *et al* (1990) Protective Activity of Tetracycline analogs against the Cytopathic Effect of the Human Immunodeficiency Viruses in CEM cells
Res. Virol. 141 5-16

Lemaitre, M., Henin, Y., Destouesse, F. *et al* (1992) Role of Mycoplasma Infection in the Cytopathic Effect induced by Human Immunodeficiency Virus Type 1 in Infected Cell Lines.
Infection and Immunity 60 742-748

Lo, S. C., Shih, J.W-X,. Yang, N.Y. *et al* (1989) A novel virus-like infectious agent in patients with AIDS.
Amer. J Trop. Med. Hyg. 41 213-226

Lo, S.C., Tsai, S., Benish, J.R. *et al* (1991) Enhancement of HIV- 1 cytocidal effects in CD4+ lymphocytes by the AIDS-associated mycoplasma
Science 251 1074-1076

Montagnier, L. and Blanchard, A (1993) Mycoplasmas as Cofactors in Infection Due to the Human Deficiency Virus
Clinical Infectious Diseases 17 309-315
Moore, J. (2002) pers comm.

Neimark, H. C. (1996) pers. comm.

Neimark, H., Barnaud, A., Gounon, P. *et al* (2002) The putative haemobartonella that influences *Plasmodium falciparum* parasitaemia in squirrel monkeys is a haemotropic mycoplasma
Microbes and Infection 4 693-698

Paton, G.R., Jacobs, J.P. and Perkins, F.T. (1965) Chromosome Changes in Human Diploid-Cell Cultures Infected with *Mycoplasma*
Nature 207 43-45

Pease, P.E., Rogers, K.B., Cole, B.C. (1967)
A cytopathogenic strain of *Mycoplasma hominis* type 1, isolated from the lung of a stillborn infant.
J Path. Bact. 94 460-462

Phillips, D. M., Pearce-Pratt, Tan X. *et al* (1992) Association of Mycoplasmas with HIV-1 and HTLV-1 in Human T Lymphocytes.
Aids Research and Human Retroviruses 8 1863-1868

Razin, S. Yogev, D. and Naot, Y. (1998) Molecular Biology and Pathogenicity of Mycoplasmas
Microbiology and Molecular Biology Reviews 62 1094-1156

Rikihisa, Y, Kawahara, M. Wen, B. *et al* (1997) Western Immunoblot Analysis of *Haemobartonella muris* Comparison of 16S rRNA Gene sequences of *H.muris, H.felis* and *Eperythrozoon suis*
J Clin.Microbiol 35 823-829

Robinson, L.B., Wickelhausen, R.H., Roizman, B. (1956) Contamination of Human Cell Cultures by Pleuropneumonia-like organisms
Science 124 1147

Stewart, S.M., Duthie, J.R., MacKay, J.M.K. *et al* (1974) Mycoplasmas and Rheumatoid Arthritis.
Ann Rheum. Dis. 33 346-352

Taylor Robinson, D. and Taylor, G (1974) Do mycoplasmas cause rheumatic disease? Symposium on Infection and Immunology in the Rheumatic Diseases ed Dumonde.
D.C. Blackwell Scientific Publications 177-186

Wildy, P.W. (1964) pers comm. Professor Wildy was the Head of the newly formed Department of Virology and Bacteriology at the time that the 'bad news' concerning mycoplasma contamination of tissue cultures was being generally understood in virological circles.

CHAPTER THREE

BACTERIAL ELEMENTS AS CRYPTO-INFECTIVE AGENTS IN HUMAN BLOOD

'It is noteworthy that HIV infection and not infection with any other agent is linked to blood transfusion associated AIDS.'

Blattner *et al* (1988)

'This statement (above) is couched in quasi-legal jargon inasmuch as it is a carefully crafted narrowly defined answer to a particular question, which is misleading in the overall impression conveyed. Such tactics may be accepted as lawyer-speak but not as the language of science'.

Pease (Chapter Eight)

INTRODUCTION 40

THE *HAEMOBARTONELLA/EPERYTHROZOON* GROUPS 40

EARLY STUDIES ON THE PARASITES IN HUMAN BLOOD 40

OBSERVATIONS ON HUMAN BLOODS 41

SIGNIFICANCE OF BLOOD BORNE BACTERIA IN HUMANS 43

MATERNAL TO FOETAL TRANSMISSION (MFT) OF MYCOPLASMAS 44

SUMMARY 44

INTRODUCTION

In the last chapter the misleading results in virological investigations caused *in vitro* by the often unsuspected presence of mycoplasmas in animal sera was emphasized. Here, the related effects of similar 'silent' infections of human serum/blood and the impact of these on laboratory and clinical studies in AIDS (discussed further in Chapter Eight) is the subject under discussion.

Much of the early work on these microorganisms in humans arose out of studies of erythrocytes of other mammals, the two main genera being *Haemobartonella* and *Eperythrozoon*. In the past, the species have been named according to the infected host, although the differences between the two genera were based on vague, arbitrary, morphological differences, which not are currently regarded as very significant. (Neimark *et al* 2001).

Recently it has been accepted that the organisms are in fact mycoplasmas - a belief held by some workers for over thirty years (see below) and this makes it clearer that the crypto-infections in human blood parallel the animal ones. The difference in their importance lies in the fact that, whereas the main problem with the crypto-infection of animal blood/serum is that these elements are likely to produce misinterpretations *in vitro*, their unsuspected presence in the blood of human patients is likely to lead to mistakes not only of interpretation *vis a vis* the relevance of HIV, but also to lead to mistakes in interpretation of the effects of therapy in AIDS patients.

THE *HAEMOBARTONELLA/EPERYTHROZOON* GROUPS

These bacteria, several of which, as explained, are now classified as mycoplasmas, are small cell-wall-less pleomorphic parasites of the erythrocytes of a wide range of animal hosts including mice, rats, cats, dogs, goats, pigs and monkeys. They are often transmitted by ectoparasites such as ticks, lice and fleas and they can also be passed from mother to foetus (see below).

They can persist for years without causing disease but in some cases clinical disease, usually including haemolytic anaemia (HA), can occur.

Splenectomy of latently infected animals often results in overt clinical disease, which usually includes HA which may be quite mild or very severe. As is the case with mycoplasma contaminated tissue cultures, treatment with tetracycline compounds can be used to eliminate infection from the infected animal.

The work that led to the final acceptance of these bacteria being mycoplasmas was based on 16S rRNA sequencing.

EARLY STUDIES ON THE PARASITES IN HUMAN BLOOD

These fall into two categories; one concerns the bacteria associated with tumours of humans and animals and is discussed in Chapter Seven; the other, concerning mycoplasmas in human blood, which arose from parallel studies on *Haemobartonella* infections of laboratory animals in Italy, and studies on the role of bacterial L-forms in rheumatoid arthritis (RA) in our laboratory, is the subject of this section.

The work on the *Haemobartonella* started in the Tedeschi laboratory, at the University of Camerino in Italy, when it was discovered that laboratory stocks of rats were infected with the agent in the absence of the ectoparasites e.g. ticks, lice and fleas commonly believed to be their vector.

Fig. 3.1 Erythrocyte Parasites in Rats (After Tedeschi *et al*)

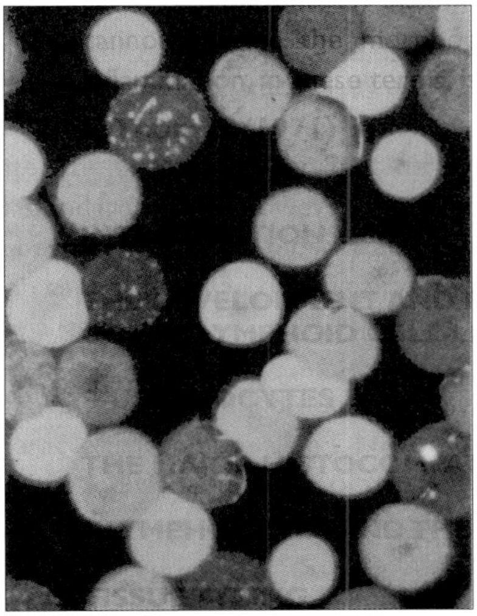

Fig. 3.1a Rat erythrocytes infected with mycoplasmas formerly known as haemobartonella

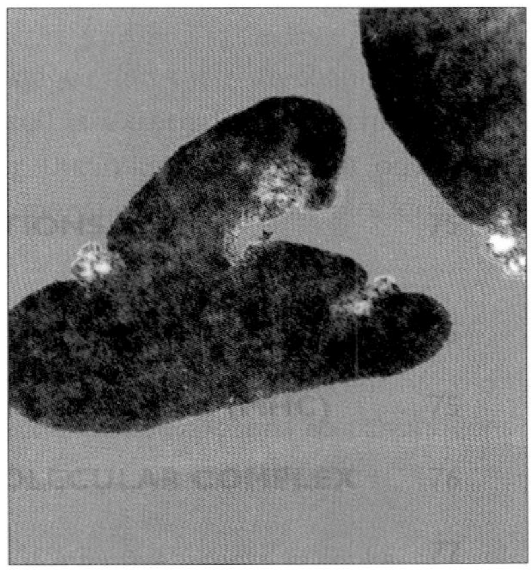

Fig. 3.1b Electron-sections showing the same as 3.1a

From the beginning of their studies the group emphasised the similarity between the haemobartonellas and the mycoplasmas, initially on morphological and histochemical grounds, and later on the similarities that exist in the life-cycles, including an intra-cellular stage, of the two groups of organisms. They found further points of similarity in the responses of the two groups of organisms to antibiotics, including resistance to tetracycline analogues and the ability of both to convert arginine to ornithine by the same metabolic pathway.

OBSERVATIONS ON HUMAN BLOODS

Tedeschi *et al* found similar haemobartonella/mycoplasma-like structures in the blood not only of human patients suffering from haemolytic disease as a result of glucose-6-phosphatase dehydrogenase deficiency and others that had undergone splenectomy for traumas, but also from the normal controls.

The group used several tecniques for the investigation of the elements, including cultural, histochemical, spectro-photometric and auto-radiological. These approaches were followed up by studies on the uptake of radioactive thymidine, uridine (Fig. 3.3) by normal erythrocytes, formate, glycine and lysine and these supported their belief that they were observing a 'diffused latent infection' which they provisionally identified as mycoplasmas.

In our laboratory, work concerning the possible role of Cell-wall-Deficient forms in RA provided support for their existence of such forms in human blood, as demonstrated by electron-microscopy (Fig. 3.2. b and c) and in experiments on the uptake of radioactive thymidine by erythrocytes of patients with RA and normal subjects (Pease 1981).

Fig. 3.2 Erythrocyte Parasites in Human Blood

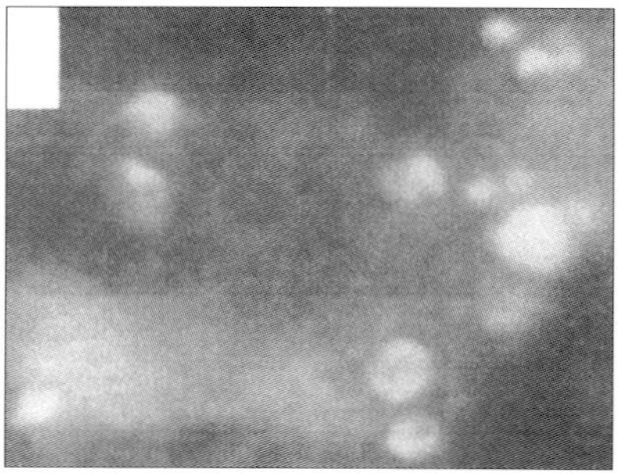

Fig. 3.2a Mycoplasma-like particles, in normal human blood, demonstrated by acridine orange staining. The green particles disappeared in the presence of Dnase - the enzyme the destroys DNA (Tedeschi *et al*)

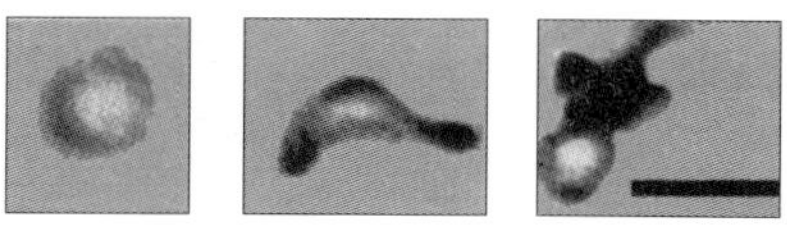

Fig. 3.2c A group of elements taken from Fig. 2b included for comparison purposes. bar=1 μm.

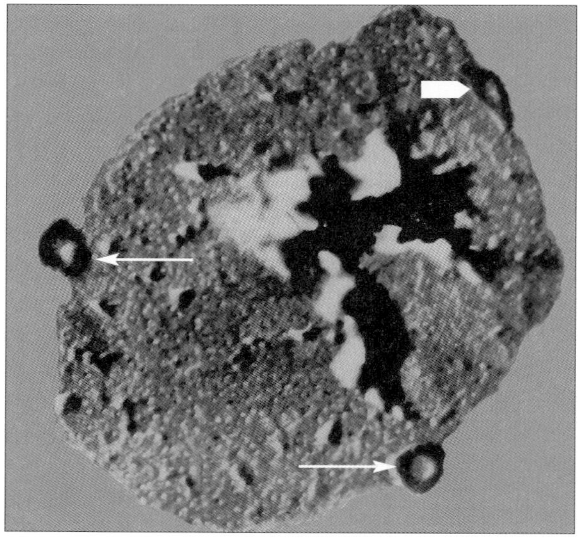

Fig. 3.2b An electron-micrograph of a normal human erythrocyte prepared in our laboratory, showing mycoplasmalike forms. Arrow-head shows a ring form starting to form filaments. Arrows show standard ringforms.

Fig. 3.3 Radioactive Studies - Uptake of Radioactive Thymidine and Uridine (After Tedeschi *et al* 1970)

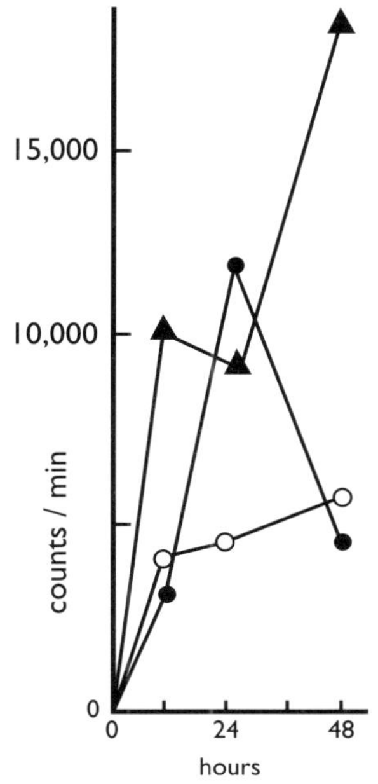

Fig. 3.3 Uptake of radioactive thymidine (DNA activity and uridine (RNA activity) by normal erythrocytes demonstrating activity on the part of the particulate matter ▲-▲ uridine; ●-● thymidineO-O thymidine at 50-fold concentration.

The incorporation of uridine was far greater than that of thymidine. After 48 hours the incorporation was still increasing, while the incorporation of thymidine reached its maximum after 24 hours and thereafter decreased.

The overall findings of the Tedeschi group concerning the incorporation of activity radioactivity were that positivity was always present from a qualitative point of view but there was considerable variation quantitatively.

In our experiments, we found that the incorporation of tritiated thymidine into cultures of erythrocytes from normal subjects and patients with RA showed that the extent of the incorporation by erythrocytes from rheumatoid patients was more variable than that by erythrocytes from normal subjects, and correlated negatively with IgG measurements and white cell counts performed on the patients' bloods, although not with the clinical activity of the patients. This suggests that the presence of the bacteria is not the prime cause of the disease and that changes in their activities are secondary to the underlying condition.

SIGNIFICANCE OF BLOOD BORNE BACTERIA IN HUMANS

As is the case with tissue contamination with mycoplasmas, their existence in human blood often goes unrecognised, and although they do not normally cause disease in healthy individuals, they are capable of causing confusion in the interpretation of result in the clinical field. Their distribution in human blood is unknown but it is quite likely to be widespread just as the equivalent micro-organisms occur in other mammals.

Haemoplasmas are likely to occur in greater numbers in immunodeficient patients than in healthy individuals since the ba lance between host and the parasite is disturbed by virtue of the defective immune system. In view of the findings of the Tedeschi laboratory and our own the possibility exists that the fluctuations of the putative HIV (Chapters Eight and Nine) in response to the 'anti-retroviral' drugs are simply due to the alterations in the RNA and to a lesser extent DNA of the unrecognised Haemoplasmas.

MATERNAL TO FOETAL TRANSMISSION(MFT) OF MYCOPLASMAS

The presence of haemoplasma/mycoplasma infection in laboratory bred animals in the absence of ectoparasite vectors showed MFT happens in animals (Amici *et al* 1966). This latter work was later confirmed in our laboratory (Bartlett and Pease 1975). This form of transmission has also been demonstrated in squirrel monkeys in captivity - in this case the investigators were able to detact *Haemobartonella* (later re-identified as a mycoplasma) on monkey foetal erythrocytes (Hugues and Michel 1999).

In humans, MFT, usually referred to as mother to child transmission (MCT) is said to occur in AIDS and as a consequence pregnant women who are sero-positive to p24 (the AIDS antigen - Chapters Eight and Nine) are being encouraged to take anti-retroviral drugs which have dangerours, even life threatening potential (afterword).

The failure to take into account the possible effects of demonstrable RNA nd DNA activity by *haemoplasma* elements, in normal human blood in this scenario can clearly be a cause of confusion in the testing for presumed HIV viral load in neonates. This along with the failure to take into account the effect of microchimerism (Chapter Nine) is extremely worrying.

SUMMARY

This is effectively a continuation of the last chapter, the emphasis being placed on the occurrence of tiny parasites, formerly known as *Haemobartonella* and *Eperythrozoon* and now recognised as mycoplasmas in the blood of animals and humans. Their presence in human and monkey blood and the implications of their going undetected in AIDS research is discussed. The potential importance of maternal to foetal transmission is also mentioned.

REFERENCES

Amici, D., Murri, O., Paparelli. *et al* (1966) Trasmissione della *Haemobartonella muris* dalla madre al feto. *Bolletino della Societa di Biologiia Sperimentale* 42 1501-1503

Bartlett, R. and Pease, P. (1975) Latent *Haemobartonella muris* infection: its transmission and decline in an inbred, ectoparasite-free strain of Wistar rat.
Parasitology 71 35-40

Hugues, C. and Michel, J-C. (1999) Haemobartonellosis in Squirrel Monkeys (Saimiri sciueus): Antagonism between *Haemobartonella* sp. and Experimental *Plasmodium falciparum* Malaria.
Exp. Parasitol. 91 297-305

Neimark, H., Johansson, K-E., Rikihisa, Y. *et al* (2001) Proposal to transfer some members of the genera *Haemobartonella* and *Eperythrozoon* to the genus *Mycoplasma* with descriptions *'Candidatus haemofaelis', 'Candidatus haemomuris', 'Candidatus haemosuis' and Candidatus wenyonii'.*
International Journal of Systematic and Evolutionary Microbiology (2001) 51 891-899

Neimark, H., Barnaud, A, Gounon, P. *et al* (2002) The putative haemobartonella that influences *Plasmodium falciparum* parasitaemia in squirrel monkeys is a haemotropic mycoplasma.
Microbes and Infection (2000) 4 693-698

Pease, P.E. (1969) Bacterial L-forms in the blood and joint fluids of arthritic subjects.
Ann. Rheum. Dis. 28 270-274

Pease, P.E. (1970) Morphological appearance of a bacterial L-form growing in association with the erythrocytes of arthritic subjects.
Ann. Rheum. Dis. 29 439

Pease, P.E. Bartlett, R. and Farr, M. (1981) Incorporation of 14C-thymidine by cultures of erythrocytes from rheumatoid arthritis patients and normal subjects, suggesting the presence of an L-form. *Experientia* 37 513-515 Birkhauser Verlag, Basel (Schweiz)

Pease, P.E. and Tallack, J. (1990) A permanent endoparasite of man; 1.The silent zoogleal /symplasm /L-form.
Microbios. 64 173-180

Rikihisa, Y. Kawahara, Wen, B. *et al* (1997) Western Immunoblot Analysis of *Haemobartonella muris* and Comparison of 16S rRNA Gene Sequences of *H.muris, H.felix,* and *Eperythrozoon suis*
J.Clin. Microbiol. 35 823-829

Tedeschi, G. G., Amici, D. and Paparelli, M. (1969) Incorporation of nucleosides and amino-acids in human erythrocyte suspensions: possible relation with a diffuse infection of mycoplasmas or bacteria in the L-form.
Nature 222 1285-1286

Tedeschi, G. G., Amici, D. and Paparelli, M. (1970) The Uptake of Radioactivity of Thymidine, Uridine, Formate, Glycine and Lysine into Cultures of Blood of Normal Human subjects: Relationship with Mycoplasma Infection.
Haematologia 4 27-47

Tedeschi, G.G. and Amici, D. (1972) Mycoplasma-like micro-organisms probably related to L-forms of bacteria in the blood of healthy persons. Cultural, morphological and histochemical data. *Annali Sclavo* 14 4

CHAPTER FOUR

INFECTION WITH ALIEN DNA - THE EXTREME CASE OF INFECTIOUS AETIOLOGY

'Great fleas have little fleas upon their backs to bite'em. And little fleas have lesser fleas and so *ad infinitum*'.

Augustus de Morgan (1872)

'Crown gall tumours can, in the light of our findings, be viewed as a feat of genetic engineering on the part of *Agrobacterium tumefaciens*.'

Chilton *et al* (1977)

INTRODUCTION	48
HISTORY	48
THE *AGROBACTERIUM/RHIZOBIUM* CONNECTION	49
GENETIC ENGINEERING, FROM THE WILD INTO THE LABORATORY AND BACK AGAIN	51
KOCH'S POSTULATES AND DNA VECTORS	52
CONCLUSION	53
SUMMARY	53

INTRODUCTION

I have previously put forward the idea that autoimmune disease in humans might represent 'the extreme case of infectious aetiology' (Pease 1965). In these disorders of the immunological system, which are discussed in Chapter Nine, the body's immune system appears to react against its own constituents and my suggestion was that tiny units of foreign DNA carried in bacteria or their sub-units could invade and colonise the cellular DNA of higher animals and humans, thereby conferring the ability of the host to produce foreign proteins, and that in the case of autoimmune diseases the body's defence mechanisms become mobilised against these substances and thus effectively against itself. In the scientific ambience of the time this was a radical viewpoint, since the received wisdom was that an insurmountable barrier existed between prokaryotic (microbial) and eukaryotic (more highly organised beings) DNA.

The first experimental evidence that this posited barrier could be breached came, a few years later, from plant biologists who discovered the genetic engineering *modus operandi* of plant cancer. Without doubt this discovery was an epoch making step forward in biology, and its impact in agriculture and medicine has been unprecedented. Although the causative agent had been known to be a bacterium, now called *Agrobacterium tumefaciens*, since 1907 when it was discovered by Erwin Smith, the actual mechanism of the loss of control of the balance between cell growth and maturation remained a mystery until the 1970's when it was realised that the actual infective agent was the 'extreme infectious agent' *i.e.* alien DNA. The source of this DNA is uncertain but several investigators believe it may have originated from a host plant in the distant past.

Another key discovery concerning a transmissible cancer-causing agent was also made in the early part of the twentieth century and this was the cause of chicken cancer. This agent, called the Rous Sarcoma Virus (RSV), was identified as a retrovirus in 1970. These viruses are the subject of the next chapter, but are mentioned here in order to introduce the idea of the essential similarity of the *modi operandi* of cancers in eukaryotes. In essence the cancer-causing capacity of retroviruses also lies in their ability to act as a vector of alien DNA - in these cases the origin is known to be the host nuclear material.

The science of genetic engineering has been developed by manipulations of these two essentially natural but disadvantageous (for the respective hosts) scenarios, and it is the purpose of this chapter to provide an introduction to the mechanism of infection by alien DNA both in the wild and in the laboratory, and thus to provide a background for the thesis which forms the basis of this book, that parallel mechanisms may be responsible for malignant and immunological disorders in humans.

HISTORY

Much of the work of Erwin Smith following his discovery of *A. tumefaciens* as the causative agent of plant cancer concerned his belief that a similar mechanism could be responsible for human cancer. It was the realisation that the galls appearing on various plants were true cancers comparable to human disease - rather than being equivalent to the granulomatous conditions, in humans, such as tuberculosis and in cattle such as 'lumpy jaw' caused by *Actinomyces* - that led him to this belief.

In his first report on the phenomenon (Smith and Townsend 1907) he described the isolation of what came to be known as *Agrobacterium tumefaciens* from the tumours (galls) that grew naturally on cultivated marguerites, sometimes called Paris daisies. The bacteria could be grown in pure culture, and tumours could be produced in other plants by inoculating them with material from the cultures with a needle. Swellings appeared within 4-5 days, were well-developed in a month and continued to grow for several months, becoming 4-5cm in diameter. Control needle inoculations with uninfected needles did not cause tumours.

Sections of the galls revealed orderly stages of transition between normal cells and fully cancerous ones, and Smith realised that 'hasty cell-division which does not allow of cell maturity proceeds in the region of inner hypertrophy until the groups of these cells are indistinguishable from the cells in the body of the tumour, either in shape, disorientation, reduction of cytoplasm, size of nucleus or affinity for stains'. He could, of course, only speculate about the nature of what later became known as the TIP (tumour inducing principle) but his suggestion that the bacteria might act after they were dead had a prophetic ring to it. The similarities between these aspects of plant and human cancers are discussed in Chapter Seven.

As far as further work in the plant cancer area was concerned, one of the first major advances in this quest was the discovery that the crown gall tumours could be maintained indefinitely *in vitro* in the absence of the bacterium (Braun 1965, also see Schell *et al* 1979 for references). Braun and his co-workers coined the expression "tumour inducing principle" (TIP) for what later proved to be the tumour inducing plasmid (pTi - see below). The TIP could transform wounded but otherwise normal plant cells into neoplastic ones, which thereafter were able to grow independently of both the bacteria and the plant, on a simple culture medium. However, it was not until the seventies that any real progress was made towards identifying the precise nature of the TIP.

THE *AGROBACTERIUM/RHIZOBIUM* CONNECTION

Fig. 4.1 Clover Nodules - a Symbiotic Relationship between Plant and Bacterium

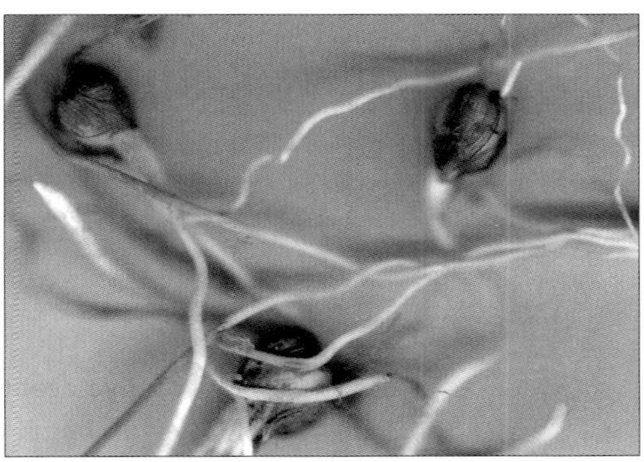

In order to put *Agrobacterium tumefaciens* in its natural context it should be explained that it belongs to the same genus as the symbiotic nitrogen-fixing bacteria known as *Rhizobium*, which are found in association with the root nodules of leguminous plants (Fig. 4.1). These are partly responsible for the high nitrogen content of these plants, to which is due the exceptional food value of peas, beans and lentils, and of lucerne and clover as animal fodder, and the use of clover as a green manure. Infection occurs shortly after the appearance of true leaves, and takes place through the root hair; a thread of bacterial growth passing up the hair into the root cortex. The root-cells are stimulated to produce a nodule, in which the bacteria multiply, and vascular strands pass into the nodule, carrying food materials, which are utilised by the bacteria. Nitrogen is fixed directly from the air by diffusion in the soil.

The symbiotic relationship between the *Rhizobium* bacterium and the plant changes when the bacterium becomes infected with a tumour-inducing plasmid (pTi). This combination results in the formation of plant tumours called crown galls. Images of crown-gall are shown in Chapter Seven.

These plasmid infected rhizobia are called agrobacteria e.g. *Agrobacterium tumefaciens* but actually the only difference between the two groups is the possession of the plasmid. This is the true cause of the cancer by virtue of its ability to upset the mechanisms controlling the relationship between cellular multiplication and maturation. The life-cycle of these bacteria is compared with the similar one of bacterial isolates from human cancer in Chapter Seven.

In our laboratory (White 1972) we studied the taxonomy of *Agrobacterium* and its close relationship to rhizobia by a computerised numerical method, technology widely acclaimed at the time, and indeed it is fair to say that this type of analysis can be useful provided that its limitations are recognised. It is helpful when very large numbers of tests involving similar biochemical mechanisms are involved, in bacteria that are already recognised as being fairly closely related. In our studies we used conventional tests in our analysis including the ability of the bacterial strains under investigation to utilize sixty-one compounds as sole carbon sources.

Our studies confirmed the idea that the genera *Agrobacterium* and *Rhizobium* should be combined, and highlighted the fact that the cancer inducing ability of some of the bacteria was the only feature that distinguished them from the rest of the group. More or less contemporaneously, work in other laboratories was leading to the conclusion that the elusive TIP, that up until that time was detectable but was not defined, was found to consist of substances that were coded for by a plasmid contained within the otherwise harmless *Rhizobium* related bacteria.

Morel and his co-workers (Petit *et al* 1970) reported the existence of two types of *A.tumefaciens* crown-gall based on their abilities to induce the synthesis of different opines in the tumours, one being octopine, and the other nopaline. Each bacterium is able not only to synthesise the particular opine, but also to use it specifically as its sole carbon and/or nitrogen source. Thus it became apparent that there is a genetic link between opine metabolism and tumour formation and that genetic information can somehow pass from bacterium to plant cell. Shortly afterwards, the Ti plasmids were discovered and their role in oncogenicity demonstrated (see Schell *el al* for references).

Work conducted subsequently by several workers allowed the mechanism of neoplastic transformation to be understood (see Chilton *et al* 1977 and 1980). These latter workers were able to demonstrate by means of DNA hybridisation experiments that crown gall tumours are caused by the incorporation of part of the Ti plasmid - the T-DNA - into the plant cells. Subsequently Chilton *el al* (1980) showed that this incorporation was, in fact, into the nuclear DNA of the plant cells (Fig.4.2)

It is now understood that the T-DNA (transferred DNA) that becomes integrated into the plant cell nucleus, codes for enzymes that synthesise the plant hormones auxin and cytokinin, which

Fig. 4.2 Diagrammatic representation of the relationship between the *A.tumefaciens* bacteria and the crown gall tumours

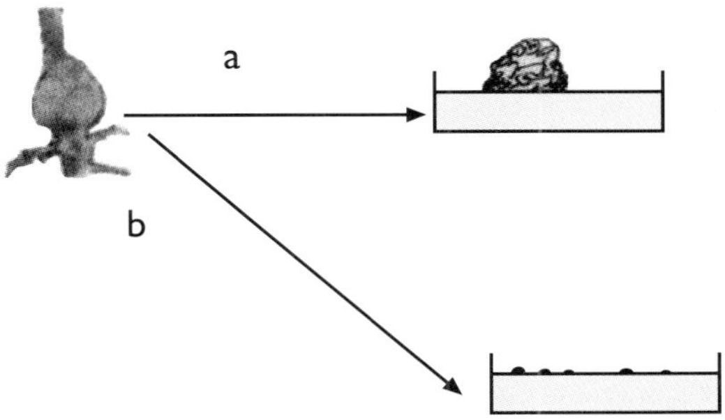

a) The tumour cells can be grown away from the plant on medium that is hormone free medium - see also Chapter Seven.

b) sub-culture of the tumour material onto nutrient agar produces colonies of *A.tumefaciens*, which can be used for infecting another plant, provided that the plant is first wounded.

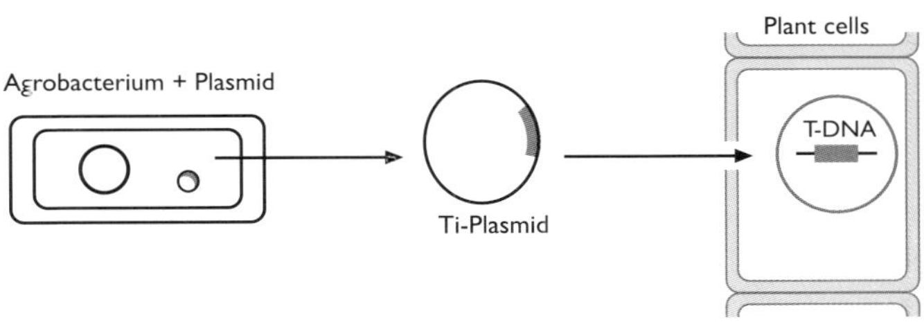

Fig. 4.3 Diagrammatic representation of the introduction of Tumour-inducing DNA (Ti plasmid) into the plant nucleus

causes the disturbance of the normal balance of plant growth control and the consequent proliferation of the undifferentiated wound tissue, which forms the crown gall. In addition the T-DNA codes for enzymes that synthesise opines and the relevant catabolic enzymes. More recent advances in this area are discussed in Chapter Seven.

GENETIC ENGINEERING FROM THE WILD INTO THE LABORATORY AND BACK AGAIN

Genetic engineering in the laboratory (LGE) took off in a spectacular way after it was discovered that it is possible to remove part of the Ti plasmid, including the tumour inducing part, and replace it with DNA of a more desirable type e.g. pesticide resistant genes from another source that could then be transferred to another plant, which is then able to express the new property.

The Ti plasmids are not suitable for use directly for this purpose, not only because of their innate cancer producing capacity, but also because they are too large to be susceptible to standard plasmid manipulation procedures, and the help of other bacterial plasmids is needed in the intermediate stages.

The classic plasmid known as pBR.322 in combination with its bacterial host *Escherichia coli* is often used in these manipulations. *E.coli* is easy to maintain and identify in the laboratory and is harmless under normal conditions. By a series of ingenious techniques it has been found possible to achieve the end result of an *Agrobacterium* carrying a disarmed vector and a donor vector that can recombine. These studies have led to the production of transgenic plants where these foreign genes can be transmitted through seeds. (Kingsman and Kingsman 1988).

In laboratory genetic engineering the processes are tightly controlled and the bacteria used to grow plasmids are disabled in such a way that escape into the general population is virtually impossible. In the wild on the other hand, bacteria are free-living agents and no comparable control exists so that transfers of DNA can occur freely. Most of these are probably abortive but when they do succeed they are often harmful to eukaryotic organisms.

On the other hand it is possible that natural genetic engineering may have had beneficial effects on evolution and *Rhizobium* might be such a case. Haemoglobin, the red pigment that carries oxygen in the blood of animals, especially chordates, also occurs in *Rhizobium*. Such a distribution might be regarded as a mere aberration of Nature, were it not for the existence in a high proportion of human erythrocytes of elements of bacteria that resemble *Rhizobium*.(Chapter Seven)

Since modern vertebrates have a much longer history than flowering plants, any transfer of genetic must have been from animal to bacterium, as in contemporary genetic engineering procedures, of which this phenomenon may be regarded as a palaeotechnic example, of great benefit to the subsequent development of mammals, which owe much to the maintenance of soil fertility by nitrogen-fixing symbiotes, as well to their food supply from, for example, clovers and lucerne: see above (Pease and Bisset 1989).

Some support comes for this from the observation that growth of tobacco plants, which are widely used in research on tumour production *via* the *Agrobacterium/Rhizobium* route, (Chapter Seven) is very considerably enhanced by the insertion of a gene coding for haemoglobin. Leif Bulow and his colleagues (Holmberg *et al* 1997) introduced the gene for bacterial haemoglobin (VHb - from *Vitreoscilla* a filamentous bacterium) into tobacco plants, and those plants that expressed the gene exhibited on average 80-100% more dry weight after 35 days of growth compared with wild type controls. Germination time was reduced from 6-8 days to 3-5 days and the growth phase from germination to flowering was 3-5 days shorter for the transgenic plants. These also contained on average 30-40% more chlorophyll and 34% more nicotine than the controls.

KOCH'S POSTULATES AND DNA VECTORS

The Postulates of Robert Koch, a pioneer German bacteriologist, who is particularly famous for his discovery of the tubercle bacillus - for which he was awarded the Nobel Prize in 1905 - have formed the basis for determining whether a specific bacterium is the cause of a particular disease.

Koch's Postulates (1890):

1) The bacteria should be found in all cases of the disease in question.

2) The bacteria should be cultured outside the body of the host, in pure culture, for several generations.

3) The bacteria, so isolated, should reproduce the disease in other susceptible animals (or plants - my addition).

4) The bacteria should then be re-isolated and again grown in artificial culture. In fact, in the case of NGE disease, these postulates can be fulfilled, with the proviso that the tumour causing DNA is the real pathogen; *A. tumefaciens* is harmless without the Ti plasmid, comparable with an unmanned troopship. The relative ubiquity of the bacteria, which at first sight would eliminate them from having an aetiological role in tumour causation, is actually a requirement, when its role is that of a vector, as opposed to being pathogenic *per se*, *i.e.* troop carriers must be readily available if the action is to be carried out.

CONCLUSION

Although the main interest in the discovery of the Ti plasmid/*Agrobacterium* package has been in its exploitation in laboratory based genetic engineering, in the present context the particular point of interest is that the alien/illegitimate DNA invasion/colonisation of the plant cells leads to tumour formation in the invaded plant, caused by the part of the integrated alien DNA that codes for enzymes that synthesise the plant hormones, auxin and cytokinin. The resulting disturbance of the normal balance between cell division and maturation with the proliferation of the undifferentiated wound tissue is reminiscent of the situation in human tumours, in which hormones and growth factors play a big part and exploitation of the normal cell mechanisms developed for wound healing also occurs.

In fact, the Chilton group themselves noted the similarity between this plant cancer and certain virus - induced animal cancers and suggested that 'it now seems reasonable to expect that some animal tumours may contain stably incorporated bacterial genes' They also expressed the opinion that the elucidation of the plant model system offered hope for the understanding of neoplastic transformation in animal cells.

Whilst the search for human cancer viruses - now called retroviruses - was pursued with great vigour, the bacterial route has not been followed to any great extent, in spite of the fact that a bacterium resembling *Agrobacterium* had already been found in association with human cancer. However, this aspect has remained quiescent and another thirty years have passed.

Although the search for a viral cause for human cancers *per se* was not successful, as will be explained in the next chapter, one of the really intriguing facts in the present context was that - as in the case of the plant cancer - a natural genetic engineering mechanism involving the transfer of growth-controlling alien DNA was found to be involved in several of the cancers of birds and mammals. The idea that the human and plant cancer have a common aetiology as proposed initially by Erwin Smith is developed in Chapter Seven.

SUMMARY

The elucidation of the discovery of the *modus operandi* of plant cancer is presented as the first demonstration of the phenomenon of natural genetic engineering (NGE) from which the whole area of laboratory and clinical discoveries, from the improvements in crops to the beginnings of gene therapy, have developed. The confirmation that the hitherto posited barrier between prokaryotic and eukaryotic DNA could be breached, with the implication that DNA can be viewed as the ultimate infective agent, is mentioned in the context of the episome theory of autoimmune disease. Brief mention is made of the techniques used in laboratory genetic engineering (LGE) in plants.

REFERENCES

Braun, A.C. (1965) The Reversal of Tumour Growth.
Sci. Am. 213 No. 5

Chilton, M-D., Drummond, M.H. Merlo, D.J. *et al* (1977) Stable Incorporation of Plasmid into Higher Plant Cells: the Molecular Basis of Crown Gall Tumourigenesis
Cell 11 263-271

Chilton, M-D, Saiki, R.K., Yadav, N. *et al* (1980) T-DNA from *Agrobacterium Ti* plasmid is in the nuclear DNA fraction of crown gall tumour cells
Proc Natl Acad Sci USA 77 4060-4064

Depicker, K, Van Montangue, M., Schell, S. (1978) Homologous DNA Sequences in different Ti plasmids are essential for oncogenicity
Nature 275 150-153

Holmberg, N., Lillius, G., and Bailey *et al* (1997) Transgenic tobacco expressing *Vitreoscilla* haemoglobin exhibits enhanced growth and altered metabolite production
Nat. Biotechnol. 15 (3) 244-247

Kingsman, S.M, Kingsman, A.J (1988) Genetic Engineering: An Introduction to Gene Analysis and Exploitation in Eukaryotes
Blackwell Scientific Publications, Oxford.

Pease, P.E. (1965) L-forms Episomes and Autoimmune Disease
E & S Livingstone Ltd., Edinburgh and London

Pease, P.E. and Bisset, K.A. (1989) Personal Discussion

Petit, A,, Delhaye, S,, Tempe J. *et al* (1970) Recherches sur les guanidines de tissus de crown gall, Mise en évidence d'une relation biochimique spécifique entre les souches de Agrobactérium et les tumeurs qu'elles induisent.
Physiol, Veg. 8 205-213

Schell W J. , Van Montagu, M., De Bruckeleer *et al* (1979) Interactions and DNA transfer between *Agrobacterium tumefaciens* and Ti-plasmid and the plant host.
Proc. R. Soc. Lond. 204 251-266

Smith. E.,F. (1911) Crown gall of Plants.
Phytopathology 1 7-11

Smith, E.F. and Townsend, O.O. (1907) A Plant Tumour of Bacterial Origin
Science 25 671-673

Smith, E. F, (1922) Appositional Growth in Crown-Gall Tumours and in Cancers.
Journal of Cancer Research 7 1-49

Virchow. R. (1871) Cellular Pathology 4th ed. Berlin as quoted by Smith E F, (1922)

White, L.O. (1972) The Taxonomy of the Crown-gall Organism Agrobacterium tumefaciens and its Relationship to Rhizobia and Other Agrobacteria
J. Gen Microbiol 72 565-574

Willmitzer, L., Beuckeleer De, Lemmers, M *et al* (1980) DNA from Ti plasmid present in nucleus and absent from plastids of crown gall plant cells
Nature 287 359-361

CHAPTER FIVE

RETROVIRUSES AS GENETIC ENGINEERS

'The hallmark of retrovirus transforming genes (*onc* genes) is specific sequences which are unrelated to essential virion genes but are closely related to sequences in normal cells'.

P. Duesberg (1983)

INTRODUCTION 58

REVERSE TRANSCRIPTASE AND THE CURRENT VIEW OF THE RETROVIRAL LIFE-CYCLE 59

RAPID TUMOUR-CAUSING *onc*-VIRUSES AS VECTORS OF EUKARYOTIC GROWTH-REGULATING GENES 60

OTHER METHODS OF DISCOVERING CELLULAR GROWTH-CONTROLLING GENES 61

HUMAN NON-*onc* RETROVIRUSES AND MALIGNANT DISEASE 62

RETROVIRUSES AND IMMUNOPATHOLOGIES - ANIMAL STUDIES 63

HUMAN RETROVIRUSES AND IMMUNOPATHOLOGIES 64

ATTEMPTED ISOLATIONS OF RETROVIRUSES FROM SJOGREN'S SYNDROME (SS) 64

RETROVIRUSES AS VECTORS IN EXPERIMENTAL STUDIES AND CLINICAL TRIALS 65

MOUSE MODELS 65

HUMAN THERAPEUTIC PROCEDURES 66

ENDOGENOUS RETROVIRUSES 66

HERV-K ACTIVITY IN MALIGNANCIES 67

HERVS IN AUTOIMMUNE DISEASES 68

THE NON-EXISTENTIALIST THEORY OF RETROVIRUSES 68

SUMMARY 69

INTRODUCTION

The concept of the retrovirus came into being in 1970 with the discovery of the enzyme reverse transcriptase (RT). Prior to that a group of agents capable of passing through filters designed to retain bacteria and which were able to cause tumours in certain avian and mammalian species had been classified as RNA tumour viruses.

What may be regarded as the prototype of this group of organisms was the first one, discovered in 1911 and known as the Rous sarcoma virus (RSV) after its discoverer. It aroused considerable interest at first, since it provided an example of an unequivocal transmissible cause of a malignancy, but chicken cancer seemed at that time unlikely to be related to human cancer and so interest faded somewhat. However, the subsequent finding of viral causes of mammalian tumours, notably in mice, led to a reconsideration of the possibility of a viral cause of human cancer, and studies on RSV were revived in the 60s. During these years, studies on RSV in particular provided background information for the further understanding of the life-cycle of the viruses.

A considerable boost to this whole line of research, based on some of these studies, was provided by the discovery of the enzyme RT, which was reported in two classic papers, published together in 1970 in *Nature*. RT is an RNA dependent DNA polymerase *i.e.* an enzyme that is able to bring about the transcription of RNA into DNA, a finding that was epoch-making at the time because it was in contradiction to the then current belief that transcription only occurred in the opposite direction.

The discovery led to the renaming of the RNA tumour viruses, including RSV, as retroviruses and then to the well-known, but unsuccessful 'War on Cancer', which was instigated in the mistaken belief that RT was exclusive to the cancer-causing viruses and accounted for their ability to bring about malignant changes.

In fact this was a wrong interpretation - RT is extremely widespread in nature and is now believed to have been in existence for millions of years and the various retro-elements - retroposons, retrotransposons and endogenous retroviruses have been present in the human genome for at least one million years.

The true cause of the ability to cause the tumours lies in the ability of the viruses to act as vectors of nearly normal gene sequences, involved in the control of growth controls, from one avian or mammalian host to another of the same species. These sequences are known as oncogenes (*oncs*) and if they are not present the ability to cause tumours is lost. This situation parallels to some extent the one that exists in plant cancer (Chapter Four).

Interest in the retroviruses faded with the failure to find an equivalent retroviral cause of human cancer until the onset of the AIDS epidemic. Once again a key discovery, in this case the finding of a particular antibody in the serum of AIDS and pre-AIDS patients, was co-opted with unseemly haste into the retroviral camp. The former cancer research workers used the techniques they had learned during the lost years of the 'War on Cancer' and research on AIDS.

It is bizarre that it is only relatively recently, twenty seven years after the launching of the concept of retroviruses, that these techniques have been validated, and have been found to be seriously wanting. These control experiments based on electron-microscope studies have demonstrated that apparently pure preparations of retro-virions have always been contaminated with cellular materials originating from the tissue cells in which they were grown.

This situation is vastly complicated by the fact that very similar sequences - including RT ones - to those accepted as being characteristic of retroviruses are found in the genes of the eukaryotic host cells in which the viruses are cultured. Some of these are referred to as endogenous retroviruses (ERVs). Thus, as in the case of contaminating mycoplasmas, discussed in Chapter Two, there is a high probability that characteristics of the contaminants - in this case of eukaryotic cell materials - have been wrongly attributed to the virus. This is of particular concern in the case of AIDS research and is discussed in detail in Chapters Eight and Nine.

It is the purpose of this chapter to provide a background to the classical views on various aspects of retrovirology, although it has proved impossible to divorce these from the relatively newly acquired information that shows that true purification of retroviruses has never been achieved.

REVERSE TRANSCRIPTASE AND THE CURRENT VIEW OF THE RETROVIRAL LIFE-CYCLE

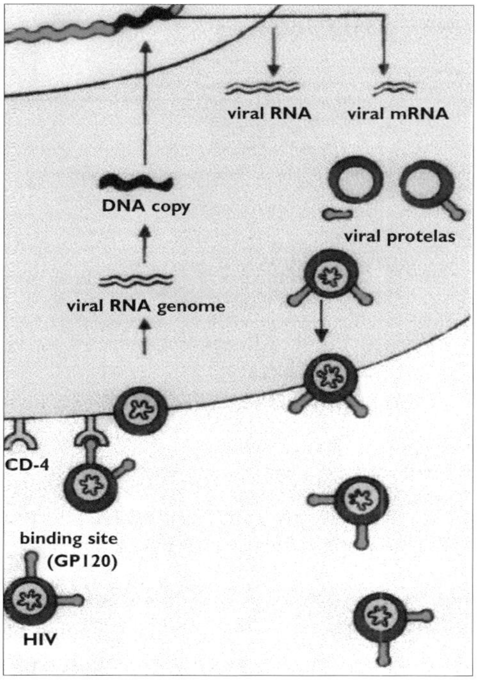

Fig. 5.1 A diagrammatic representation of the life-cycle of retroviruses (After Williams *et al* 1989)

At the time of the publications on RT by Temin and Baltimore in 1970, it was generally recognised that in the multiplication and transformation of cells, RSV needs the synthesis of a new DNA different from that produced in the cell during the S phase (the stage in the cell cycle where there is much activity, particularly in the synthesis of DNA) and specific for the virus. Since RSV was regarded as purely an RNA virus both authors reasoned that an enzyme that would synthesise DNA from RNA might be present in the virions. Actually, Baltimore's main observations were made on a mouse leukaemia virus (Rauscher mouse leukaemia virus) but the results were in agreement.

The techniques used were simple ones. The viral particles were (allegedly) separated from the cells and tested for their ability to take up radioactive thymidine so demonstrating the formation of DNA. The resulting product was characterised as DNA and the fact that RNA was the template was confirmed by the demonstration that uptake of the thymidine was inhibited by pancreatic ribonuclease.

This discovery of RT led to the elucidation of the life-cycle of retroviruses including their DNA stage.

The critical property of the viruses in the present context is believed to be vested in their ability to integrate into the cellular DNA of the host. This is achieved by the capacity of their double stranded DNA, transcribed from their RNA by reverse transcriptase, to circularise and integrate into host DNA and produce what is called the proviral form, which is, in effect, a genetic parasite.

It becomes permanently integrated (named provirus) in the chromosomal DNA, where it is replicated during the cell-cycle like cellular genes are and then passed to daughter cells. This is the property that makes retroviruses able to introduce foreign genes into eukaryotic cells thus conferring a permanent change on these cells, which in the wild may cause cancer or in the laboratory by suitable manipulation of the system may be used for a range of experimental studies e.g. for the determination of the steps in haemopoiesis and in clinical trials in gene therapy.

During replication, RNA transcripts are produced from proviral DNA and are transported to the cell cytoplasm where they can be translated into viral proteins. Viral precursor structural proteins and replication assemble with viral RNA to form new virion cores and these are released from cells by budding through the plasma membrane where they acquire a membrane envelope where the viral *env* proteins (see below) are embedded. This budding process does not kill the cells and they can go on producing viruses over long periods.

RAPID TUMOUR-CAUSING *onc*-VIRUSES AS VECTORS OF EUKARYOTIC GROWTH-REGULATING GENES

Retroviruses contain three main genes - gag pol env - the gag encodes for the internal core structure, the pol for RT and the env for the envelope proteins. In addition there are long terminal repeats (LTRs) which contain non-coding sequences containing regulatory, i.e. promoter and enhancer, elements for viral gene expression.

Some retroviruses cause the rapid unequivocal onset a short time after infection and these are the ones that contain cancer-causing genes - oncogenes (oncs). Essentially these are sequences that originate in the actual eukaryotic host cell nuclei e.g. of the chicken or the mouse. These cancer causing genes (oncs) carried by the cancer-causing retroviruses and called v-onc genes consist of hybrids between traduced (kidnapped) host genes and viral genes.

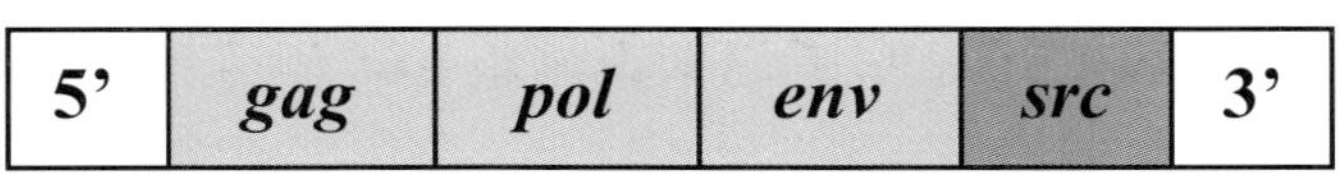

Fig. 5.2a The structure of the Rous Sarcoma Virus (RSV) – this particular retrovirus contains all the genes necessary for replication as well as the chicken DNA that causes the malignancy

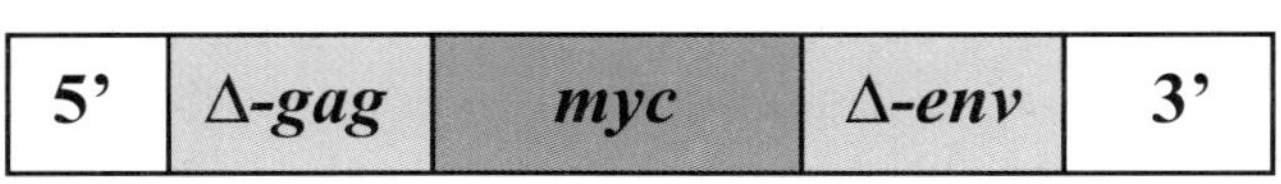

Fig. 5.2b The structure of the Avian Myelocytomatosis virus (MC29)

Much effort has been expended in attempts to identify the proteins encoded by these genes and to discover how they bring about malignant changes. The *v-onc* product activities are almost all concerned with growth control mechanisms, which when carried into the DNA of the new host perturb the regulation of several factors, especially growth promoting hormones breaks down and the progression towards cancer is initiated.

There are several similar retroviruses of birds and some mammals that contain oncogenes (*oncs*), which are capable of causing a variety of malignancies. By the use of hybridisation and nuclear sequencing techniques about thirty *v-onc* genes have now been revealed. The extent of the virus gene deletion or truncation and the position of the also sometimes truncated proto-oncogene derived *v-onc* part vary from isolate to isolate. Each of the *oncs* has been given a different name, three letters in italics based on the name of the virus from which it was isolated.

The labelling of the genes is rather confusing and needs a word of explanation. It is a facet of scientific research that during the course of investigations workers need to label the things they are investigating and sometimes, as is inevitable in research, mistakes in interpretations are made and concepts have to be altered.

In cancer research it was originally believed that certain cellular genes were actually cancer-causing *per se* and these became known as cancer-causing or oncogenes. It was thought that oncogenes had been deposited in the human genome by some sort of genetic accident that occurred in the distant past. In reality these genes are normal regulatory ones that when disturbed by outside influences may lose their ability to control the connection between cell division and maturation, thus leading to cancer.

Misleadingly the normal cellular growth controlling genes are now referred to as proto-oncogenes and the term *onc* is still used in referring to the transduced normal genes carried by the retrovirus vectors.

The similarity of the retrovirus/*onc* scenario to the *Agrobacterium*/*Ti* one already mentioned, lies in the infective agent - the extreme case of an infective aetiology (Pease 1965) - which is alien DNA and whilst there is some question about the origin of the T-DNA in crown gall tumour formation, there is no doubt that in the retrovirus scenario the cancer-causing DNA has been derived from another *host of the same species*. Thus certain microorganisms acting as vectors for DNA are able to breach the integrity of the body (Chapters Six and Nine) at a clonal level so that the DNA from one individual can invade the cell control mechanisms of another, thus providing the potential for malignant and autoimmune disease.

OTHER METHODS OF DISCOVERING CELLULAR GROWTH-CONTROLLING GENES

Whilst the study of the *onc*-retroviruses has led to the identification of the detection of some thirty *onc* genes, studies on actual tumour material have led to the discovery of at least fifty more. One of the means of investigation has been by studies on gene transfer usually called DNA transfection - the most used cells in this are cultures of a mouse embryo fibroblast line, NIH/3T3.

The use of this procedure resulted from a classic experiment in which cells from a human bladder tumour were introduced into NIH-3T3 cells and after several weeks the cultures showed transformed cells due, in this case, to the introduction of an oncogene which on analysis proved to be related to the retroviral *ras* genes.

Other genes associated with cancer have been discovered by this technique and also by observations on non-*onc* retroviruses and by the study of chromosome abnormalities (Chapter Seven).

HUMAN NON-*onc* RETROVIRUSES AND MALIGNANT DISEASE

The search for human cancer-causing retroviruses was frustrating from the start and although there were several reports of successful isolations from human sources most proved to be caused by contamination of tissue cultures with monkey viruses. Eventually a human retrovirus was identified in the Gallo laboratory in 1980 (Poiesz *et al*).

This virus, now known as the Human T-cell leukaemia virus (HTLV-1), was found in two cell-lines established from a patient with a T-cell lymphoma (*mycosis fungoides*) as well as from the patient's fresh peripheral blood lymphocytes. Eventually a connection of sorts was detected between it and a type of adult T-cell leukaemia that occurs in inhabitants of the Japanese island of Kyushu, in some parts of Africa and in the Caribbean, which led Gallo to believe that he had isolated the causative agent of that type of leukaemia. However the connection is regarded by several authorities as being very tenuous.

Clearly since HTLV-1 does not contain an *onc*-gene comparable to the v-*oncs* just described- it is known as a non-*onc* virus - its role and that of other non-*onc* retroviruses in cancer-causation, if any, is not the same. There have been some suggestions that the insertion of retrovirus promoter elements close to cellular regulatory genes e.g. *myc* could act as 'illegitimate' collaborators so that *myc* is over-expressed thus leading to excessive cellular growth, which could eventually lead to cancer (Teich 1991).

However, Duesberg (1987 and 1987a) presented a good case for the belief that generally speaking, except for retrovirus infections of very young animals or animals under special conditions in the laboratory, retroviruses, including HTLV-1 are relatively non-pathogenic and any connection with malignant transformation rests in their tendency to cause hyperplasia, thus providing a suitable background for transformation caused by something else. His views on aneuploidy being sufficient to cause cancer are discussed in Chapter Seven.

The main points of relevance in his arguments are that first, the percentage of symptomatic carriers is very low, and second, that the latent periods that exist between infection with e.g. HTLV-1 are usually very long *i.e.* ten to over thirty years - compared with a few days in the case of the onc viruses. Duesberg also raised these two points with respect to HIV and AIDS in the 1987 paper, which included his first major criticism of the HIV equals AIDS concept.

RETROVIRUSES AND IMMUNOPATHOLOGIES - ANIMAL STUDIES

The first well-known association of retroviruses with immunopathology was discovered in New Zealand Black (NZB) mice, which are particularly prone to immunological deficiencies. They were bred in Dunedin New Zealand during experiments designed to produce black mice from wild mice that had originally been captured in England. The resulting NZB mice develop a wide variety of tolerance defects leading to autoimmune haemolytic anaemia and/or glomerulonephritis and some develop malignant lymphomas.

Fig. 5.3 Virus-like Particles in New Zealand Black Mice

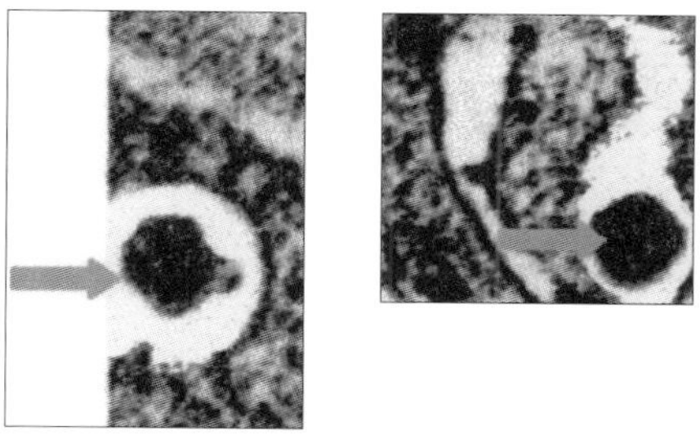

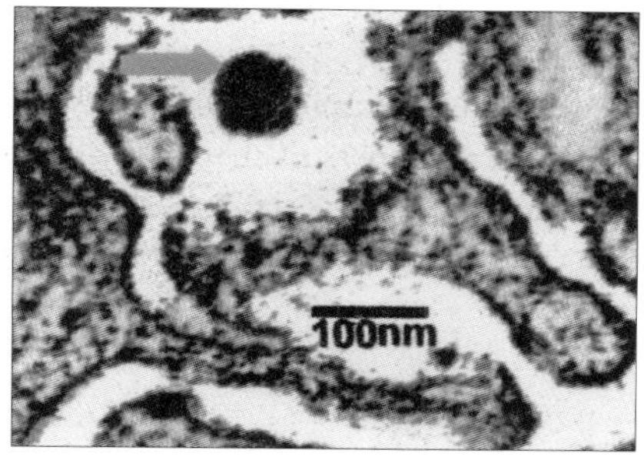

Fig. 5.3 Electron-sections of NZB mouse kidneys showing virus-like particles (arrows)

The discovery of ultra-structurally virus-like particles, later identified as type C retroviruses, from NZB mice (Mellors and Huang 1966, Mellors 1967) initially gave the impression that there was a cause and effect relationship between the retrovirus and the immunodeficiency and lymphoma production. Type 'C' murine oncogenic virus-like particles were shown to be present in distinct places, notably in kidney tubules of new-born NZB mice, old NZB mice, some NZB hybrid mice and Swiss mice inoculated with NZB spleen cell-free filtrate.

However, the high hopes that the cause of some types of immune-deficiency diseases and even malignant disorders had been found were dashed with the discovery, based on the examination of the progeny of crosses between NZB mice and a strain of normal white mice (SWR) that retrovirus expression was not needed for the development of the immunodeficiency. The dissociation between virus expression and the development of immune pathology was not peculiar to NZB X SWR crosses, similar results were found in NZB and other normal mice.

These results add weight to the possibility that the HIV/AIDS connection is not causative and other mouse models of human immunopathologies such as those for Systemic Lupus Erythematosis (SLE), and allo-immune mice (Chapter Eight) add further support to the non-role of retroviruses in immunopathologies. Similarly experiments with vaccines developed in the course of the search for an AIDS prevention program, performed on the macaques, also support the view that HIV and AIDS are separate entities (Chapter Nine).

Several reviews on the subject of retroviruses and autoimmunities e.g. (Garry *et al* 1995) refer to naturally occurring diseases associated with retroviruses in animals with the implication that they provide models for the human diseases. The two most often mentioned being caprine arthritis-encephalitis virus (CAEV), which is believed to cause arthritis in some adult goats and is regarded as a valuable model for human rheumatoid arthritis (RA) and the Ovine Maedi/Visna virus associated with interstitial pneumonia in sheep, which has been claimed to be an animal model for one of the common complications in human SLE and paediatric AIDS. This is an area where more research is needed with special emphasis on the elimination of mycoplasmas as causative agents in these conditions.

HUMAN RETROVIRUSES AND IMMUNOPATHOLOGIES

Currently the most important field of study in this area is in HIV/AIDS, but since there is such a vast amount of information available, out of all proportion to that on the classic immunopathologies, this has been accorded a Chapter of its own (Chapter Eight). However certain aspects about AIDS need to be mentioned here in order to understand the perspective of viewing AIDS as essentially an immunopathology with much in common with Systemic Lupus Erythematosis (SLE) and related conditions (see Appendix One for a brief description of these).

The concept of HIV as the cause of AIDS was originally based on the belief that sero-positivity to the 'AIDS' antigens p24 and gp120 was elicited by a specific infective agent. The possibility that they were responses to altered self-antigens was not considered even though the condition is characterised by the production of autoantibodies to an extent comparable to that found in SLE and that AIDS is clearly a disorder of the immune system.

The HIV work on AIDS initially led to hopes that retroviruses could be the answer to the other immunological disorders and the interesting point is that although sero-positivity to these antigens was demonstrated - both in the SLE mice (p24 and gp120) and humans (p24) in 30% of SLE patients and other disorders - no corresponding retrovirus has been found.

In other words, whilst these antibodies are characteristic of immuno-pathologies their occurrence and consequent efficacy as diagnostic indicators does not *per se* imply the involvement of a retrovirus. These points are discussed at greater length in Chapters Eight and Nine.

ATTEMPTED ISOLATIONS OF RETROVIRUSES FROM SJOGREN'S SYNDROME (SS)

The most widely quoted report on this subject was published by Garry *et al* (1990) who identified virus-like particles, which they named Human Intracisternal A Retrovirus (HIAP), in H9 cells that had been cultured with salivary gland tissue from SS patients. The particles separated out on a sucrose gradient at 1.22g ml and this fraction also contained RT activity and material that reacted with antibody to p24. However no aetiological relationship has been proved.

Stimulated by the work of the Garry group, Griffiths *et al* (1997) investigated the expression of retrovirus sequences in SS. and detected novel sequences spanning parts of a retrovirus in eight individuals. They failed to find similar sequences in uninfected human cell-lines indicating what they considered to be a hitherto unrecognised infectious retrovirus (HRV-5). However they were unable to connect them with the aetiology of SS.

Interest in the possibility of retroviral involvement in both malignant and immuno-pathological diseases has now moved on to studies on endogenous retroviruses; see below.

RETROVIRUSES AS VECTORS IN EXPERIMENTAL STUDIES AND CLINICAL TRIALS

The successful redirecting of the cancer-causing potential of the *Ti* plasmid carried by *Agrobacterium tumefaciens* into the beneficial channels of improving crops paved the way towards what is now called gene therapy. The aim is to prepare retrovirus vectors that could deliver a gene to a target eukaryotic cell taking advantage of the same *modus operandi* as the *onc*-virus that occurs in nature.

The hope is that this technique might in the long run provide treatment for inherited diseases such as Huntington's chorea, cystic fibrosis, and severe inherited immunodeficiency disease (SCID), and eventually for cancer and arthritis.

MOUSE MODELS

In the simplest type, the retroviral provirus DNA is treated so that most of the replicative *gag pol* and *env* genes are removed, leaving the regions needed for replication, integration and RNA synthesis intact. This region is replaced by the gene intended for transfer and also a selectable gene, one whose presence in transformed cells is readily detectable, thus marking out the cells that have been transformed.

The resulting proviruses (plasmids) are propagated in *E coli* in a way analogous to the propagation of plasmids such as the *Ti* one in the wild and more directly to the manipulated Ti in pBR.322 in the laboratory described in Chapter Four. After the propagation, the DNA is used to transfect a suitable cell line such as NIH 3T3 and here the marker gene indicates the location of the transformed cells. These virus producing cells are then co-cultivated with bone marrow cells from mice previously treated with a chemical (5-fluorouracil (5-Fu)) which allows enrichment of primitive precursor cells. (Fig. 5.6).

Studies of this kind have shown that up to eighty-five per cent of primitive stem cells can be transformed with retrovirus vectors and that when antibiotic resistant cells from the spleen of the reconstituted mice are injected into secondary recipients the whole haematopoietic system of these recipients can become reconstituted. Cells of all lineages isolated from the secondary recipients are resistant to the antibiotic, showing that cells capable of self renewal have been transformed.

These studies in fact provide a good model of how infection with vector borne alien DNA in human marrow cells could give rise to human malignant and immunological pathologies (Chapters Seven and Nine).

Fig. 5.4 Manipulation of Pluripotent Haematopoietic Stem Cells

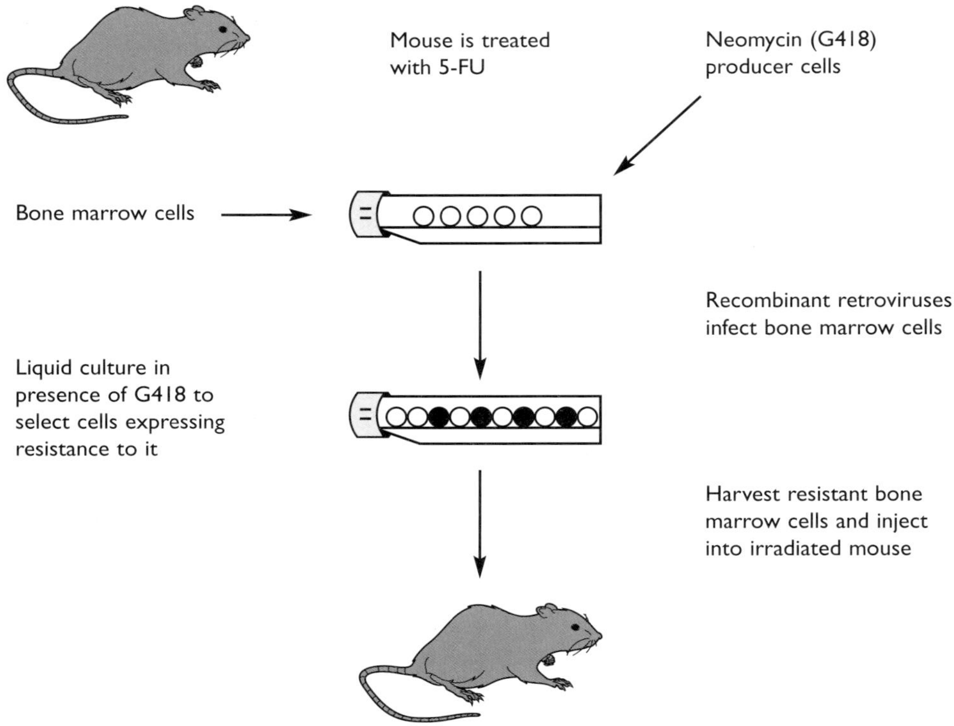

HUMAN THERAPEUTIC PROCEDURES

In human gene therapy the idea is to remove bone marrow cells from the patient, manipulate these *in vitro*, introducing a wild type gene to replace a defective gene, by means of a retroviral vector, and to return the cells to the patient.

There is obviously a long way to go before these hopes can be realised and there are vast ethical and financial aspects as well as technical problems that need to be taken into account and these are well outside the scope of this book. Recent trials have had to be halted because patients, who at first showed some improvement, have become seriously ill afterwards. Complications, it is suggested, arise from the presence in the patients of endogenous retroviruses and alternative vectors are now being sought.

ENDOGENOUS RETROVIRUSES

The fact that nucleotide sequences, which were regarded as characteristic of RSV, avian leucosis and mammalian leukaemia viruses, were also present in the uninfected cells of their respective hosts was known as early as 1966 but it was not recognised as ambiguous.

Standard practice would have been to resolve this ambiguity by electron-microscopy of the preparations and a scrutiny of the purification techniques to validate these, so eliminating the obvious possibility that the sequences were not those of the virus but only of the host cells in which they were grown. No such tests were performed and the legacy of this bizarre omission remains with us until this day.

Such, however, was the *idée fixe* concerning the idea that RT = retrovirus = cancer in the early days, that the idea that cellular elements might be contributing to the results obtained by the investigations of 'purified' virions was ignored. We now know that these eukaryotic cells not only contain the nucleotide sequences supposed to exist also in the 'virions' but also ones for RT. In fact it is now realised that apparently pure preparations of retrovirus virions often consist of considerably more cellular material than of virus-like particles.

In fact it now seems possible that the sidetracking of the discovery of RT into the narrow field of unproductive retrovirus/cancer research impeded the recognition of its potentially great importance in biology as a whole. Interest in the possible role of retroelements in evolution and in the regulatory and repair processes in individual cells has been considerably stimulated by the sequencing of the human genome - the human genome project - but so far there are only inklings of the mechanisms involved.

The project has indicated that about eight per cent of the human genome consists of retro-elements, and that some of these resemble the classic retrovirus structure (see above) so closely, that they are called human endogenous retroviruses (HERVs).

These are classified into three main categories corresponding roughly to the animal virus ones. However, the only ones that need concern us here are the Class II ones which are referred to as HERV-Ks, and which are regarded as homologues of the Mammary Mouse Tumour Virus (MMTV). HERV-Ks, of which it is now understood there are twenty-five to fifty copies in the human genome, sometimes occur in an intact or almost intact form (Mayer *et al*, 1999, Reus *et al* 2002). Furthermore, HERV-Ks are among those HERVs which often become activated in patients with malignant and immunological diseases.

Such activation of the cells may result in the production of proteins, not normally recognised by the immune system of the host, with the consequent production of autoantibodies. Virus-like particles resembling stages in the presumed life-cycle of retroviruses may be produced accompanied by RT activity.

HERV-K ACTIVITY IN MALIGNANCIES

There are several reports of some HERV-Ks giving rise to virus-like particles, associated with RT activity, in human mammary tumours and from human mammary carcinoma-derived cell-lines.

Ono *et al* (1987) investigated the expression of HERV-K in human tumour cell cultures and found it to be expressed in several cell-lines and of particular interest was their finding that its expression in the breast cell-line T47D mentioned above was under hormonal control.

Later studies by Patience *et al* (1996) on the cell-line T47D confirmed that the cells produce virus-like particles that band at the typical density for retroviral particles on a sucrose gradient, possess RT activity and package HERV-K10-like sequences. In addition they identified open reading frames, which could encode the RT and RNase H (this degrades the RNA template after it has been copied).

Testicular tumour cell-lines derived from embryonic carcinomas or teratocarcinomas have also provided some interesting relevant facts. These lines produce particles which are known as human teratocarcinoma derived virus particles (HDTVs).

HERVS IN AUTO-IMMUNE DISEASES

In addition to the retrovirus like properties already mentioned, HDTV/HERV-K is capable of eliciting the formation of antibodies in certain disease conditions and the fact that there is a decline in these titres following tumour removal suggests that the increased HERV activity was a result of the condition rather than the cause (Boller *et al* 1997). Similar observations have been made with respect to the occurrence of transient sero-positivity to the p24 'AIDS' antigen in patients that have received therapeutic transplants. In both these cases it seems that the antibodies were in fact autoantibodies (Chapter Nine).

Some more recent work supports the interpretation that that HERV activation. For example in a study into the augmentation of the expression of four HERV families in human monocytes and autopsied brain tissue from patients with inflammatory brain disease, Johnston *et al* (2001) suggested that the increased expression of the HERV activity was a consequence of increased immune activity rather than the cause of the diseases. In a similar vein Obermayer-Staub and Manns (2001) queried whether HERVs are aetiological agents of autoimmune diseases or an epiphenomenon, induced by inflammatory processes - (possibly induced by a co-infecting virus).

Clearly the study of ERVs and their role in human and animal disease is in its infancy and much more work is required before their significance is truly understood. Roswitha Lower (1999) has provided an excellent review of the various facets of endogenous retroviruses, including; their pathogenic potential via insertional mutations and recombinations; their possible protective effects against exogenous retrovirus infections, and of foetuses and the problems of their possible effects in gene therapy and xenotransplantation.

THE NON-EXISTENTIALIST THEORY OF RETROVIRUSES

It is believed by some investigators that the presumed exogenous retrovirus activities are in fact due to ERV activity combined with the activity of unrecognised bacterial elements especially mycoplasmas. As explained above, the cells used to culture these retroviruses are the ones most likely to have heightened activation of their endogenous retroviruses (this applies also to foetal/neonatal material). This activation manifests itself by the production of virus-like particles and RT activity. This combined with the activities of bacterial/mycoplasma elements - which are often close in size to the putative retroviruses - especially cytopathogenicity could be an alternative explanation for the whole concept of retrovirology. These aspects are discussed further in Chapters Eight and Nine.

SUMMARY

This chapter is intended to provide background information about retrovirology. The history of the discovery of RT and the consequent renaming of the RNA tumour viruses as retroviruses and their proposed life-cycles, involving DNA and RNA, is described. The role of retroviruses as pathogens in the malignancies and in the immunopathologies is discussed and it is pointed out that the evidence, including animal studies, for them being aetiological agents *per se* is not robust. AIDS is mentioned in the context of its being an immunopathology and it is indicated that the belated finding that cellular material has never been separated from the virions casts a shadow, not only on AIDS research, but also over retrovirology as a whole. Endogenous retroviruses are discussed both in the light of their potential confusion with exogenous viruses and in their possible involvement in human disease. Genetic experiments in mice using retroviruses vectors with the object of paving the way to gene-therapy in humans are discussed, mainly in the context of how these laboratory experiments give indications of how alien DNA transfers exist in the wild, leading to human diseases as discussed in later chapters.

REFERENCES

Baltimore, D (1970) RNA-dependent DNA Polymerase in Virions of RNA Tumour Viruses
Nature 226 1209-1211

Baltimore, D (1976). Viruses, Polymerases and Cancer
Science 192 632-636

Bittner, J.J. (1942) The milk-influence of breast tumours in mice.
Science 95 462-463

Boller, K., Janssen, O., Schuldes, H. *et al* (1997) Characterisation of the Antibody Specific response for the Human Endogenous Retrovirus HTDV/HERV-K.
J. Virol. 71 4581-4588

Datta, S. K. (1988) Murine Lupus
Methods in Enzymology 162 384-412

Duesberg, P.H. (1983) Retroviral transforming genes in normal cells?
Nature 304 219-26

Duesberg, P.H. (1987) Retroviruses as Carcinogens. Expectations and Reality
Perspectives in Cancer Research. 47 1199-1220

Duesberg, P.H. (1987a) Cancer genes: Rare recombinants instead of activated oncogenes (A Review). *Proc. Natl. Acad. Sci. U.S.A.* 84 217-224

Garry, R. F., Fermin, C.D., Hart, D.J. *et al* (1990) Detection of a Human Intracisternal A-Type Retroviral Particle Antigenically Related to HIV
Science 250 1127-1129

Garry, R.F., Kreig, A.M., Cheevers, W.P. (1995) Retroviruses and Their Roles in Chronic Inflammatory Diseases and Autoimmunity
The Retroviridae 4 491-602

Griffiths, D.J., Venables, P.J., Weiss, R.A. *et al* (1997) A novel exogenous retrovirus sequence identified in humans.
J. Virol. 71 2866-2872

Griffiths, D.J. (2001) Endogenous retroviruses in the human genome sequence
Genome Biol. 2 1017.1-1017.5

Johnston, J.B., Silva, C., Warren, K.G. *et al* (2001) Monocyte activation and differentiation augment human endogenous retrovirus expression: implications for inflammatory brain diseases
Ann. Neurol. 50 429-430

Kingsman, S. J. and Kingsman. A. J. (1990) Genetic Engineering.
Blackwell Scientific Publications. Oxford, London, Edinburgh.

Lower, R. (1999) The pathogenic potential of endogenous retroviruses: facts and fantasies
Trends in Microbiology 7 350-356

Lower, R., Boller, K., Hasenmaier, B. *et al* (1993) Identification of human endogenous retroviruses with complex mRNA expression and particle formation
Proc. Natl. Acad. Sci. 90 4480-4484

Lower, R, Lower, J. and Kurth, R. (1996) The viruses in all of us: Characteristics and biological significance of human retrovirus sequences
Proc.Natl.Acad.Sci. 93 5177-5184

Mayer, J., Sauter, M., Racz, *et al* (1999) An almost-intact human endogenous retrovirus K on chromosome 7
Nature genetics 21 257-258

Mellors, R., C. and Huang, C.Y. (1966) Immunopathology of NZB/Bl mice. V. Virus-like (filterable) agent separable from lymphoma cells and identifiable by electron-microscopy.
J. Exptl. Med 124 1031

Mellors, R. C. and Huang, C.Y. (1967) Immunopathology of NZB/Bl Mice VI. Virus separable from Spleen and Pathogenic for Swiss Mice *J. Exptl. Med* 126 53-62

Ono, M., Kawakami,M. and Ushikubo, H. (1987) Stimulation of expression of the human retrovirus genome by female steroid hormones in human breast cancer cell line T47D
J.Virol 61 2059-2062

Orenstein, J.M. (2000) Isn't a Picture Still worth a thousand Words?
Ultrastructural Pathology 24 67-74

Patience, C., Simpson, G.R., Colletta, A.A. *et al* (1996) Human Endogenous Retrovirus Expression and Reverse Transcriptase Activity in the T47D Mammary Carcinoma Cell Line.
J.Virol. 70 2654-2657

Poiesz, B.J., Ruscetti, F.W., Gadzar, A.F. *et al* (1980) Detection and isolation of type C retrovirus particles from fresh and cultured lymphocytes of a patient with cutaneous T-cell lymphoma
Proc. Natl.Acad.Sci. USA 77 7415-7419

Reus, K., Mayer, J. Sauter, M. *et al* (2001) Genomic Organisation of the Human Endogenous Retrovirus HERV-K(HML-2.HOM) (ERVK6) on Chromosome 7
Genomics 72 314-320

Teich, N,M. (1991) Oncogenes and cancer in Introduction to the Cellular and Molecular Biology of Cancer 2nd edition eds L.M. Franks and N.M. Teich

Temin, H and Mitzutani (1970) RNA-dependent DNA polymerase in of Rous Sarcoma Virus
Nature 226 1211-1214

Wiliams, I., Mindel, A. and Weller, V.D. (1989) AIDS Gower Medical Publishing London and New York

CHAPTER SIX

IMMUNOLOGICAL ASPECTS

'Without these (defence mechanisms) I have no doubt that life on earth would eventually become a kind of flowing syncitium in which I cannot imagine the morphogenesis of a flower. The opposite of inflammation, in these terms, is symbiosis'.

L. Thomas (1971)

INTRODUCTION	74
THE DEVELOPMENT AND FUNCTIONS OF THE LYMPHOID CELL-LINES	75
B-LYMPHOCYTES	75
THE MAJOR HISTOCOMPATIBILITY COMPLEX (MHC)	75
T-LYMPHOCYTES AND THE TRIMOLECULAR COMPLEX	76
TISSUE TYPING	77
THE COMPLEMENT SYSTEM	77
SUPERANTIGENS	78
THE HLA-B27 CONNECTION WITH THE SPONDYLOARTHROPATHIES	78
GRAFT VERSUS HOST REACTIONS IN CHIMERAS	79
BENIGN CHIMERISM	80
GRAFT VERSUS HOST DISEASE - DISEASE-CAUSING CHIMERISM	80
HETEROPHILE ANTIBODIES	81
THE WEIL-FELIX REACTION	82
MOLECULAR MIMICRY AND RHEUMATIC FEVER	83
SUMMARY	83

INTRODUCTION

Immunology, which is basically the study of the body's mechanisms for recognising and destroying invading microorganisms, became a discipline in its own right during the nineteen sixties. At that time great efforts were made to solve the problems of the immunological pathologies such as rheumatoid arthritis, and several new immunological techniques were developed in pursuit of that aim. Up until then, immunology was employed mainly for the diagnosis of bacterial infections, and later for classifying bacteria.

One of the simplest of these immunological diagnostic techniques is the agglutination of bacteria in the presence of their specific antisera. In the case of a bacterial infection e.g. typhoid fever, patients develop antibodies to the bacterium in their blood serum, which when separated from the other blood components reacts specifically with suspensions of the bacteria on a slide or in a test tube (*in vitro*) causing them to form clumps visible to the naked eye.

The highest dilution of serum at which agglutination still occurs is known as the titre of antibodies present and if this titre increased over a period of days the diagnosis of typhoid fever could be made. The detection of this 'rising titre' became even more critical after the introduction of vaccination against typhoid because the procedure causes the production of homologous protective antibody to *S.typhi* in healthy individuals.

Considerable advances have been made in immunology since the time when it was effectively a subsection of bacteriology. Progress was made in the fields of the elucidation of the development and functions of the B and T-cell lymphocytes; in the discovery and characterisation of the human histocompatability (Human Leukocyte Antigen-HLA) system; in the understanding of the phenomena of graft rejection and graft versus host disease (GVHD) and in the association of certain HLA types with particular diseases.

There is no doubt that some of these developments have improved the prospects in the field of organ transplantation in humans very considerably and realisation of the hopes for successful gene therapy in some areas seems to be finally within reach. However, the immunopathologies are still not really understood (Chapter Nine) and in particular the HLA-disease connection (see below), although definite and very strong indeed in the classic ankylosing spondylitis/HLA-B27 association, still remains in the minds of many workers something of a mystery.

Attempts have often been made to identify causative agents of various immunopathologies by searching for antibodies to infective agents in patients' sera in spite of the fact that results are likely to be prejudiced because of damage to the immune system. If these approaches are not treated with caution and in the context of clinical factors, they can lead to errors of interpretation. This is particularly likely to happen in the so-called autoimmune diseases, in which the body appears to react against its own components. In these conditions there is likely to be a considerable overlap in the range of antibodies in the patients' sera, and it is important not to confuse these with reactions to exogenous (outside) infective agents. In Chapters Eight and Nine the possibility that the occurrence of specific antibody patterns that are diagnostic for AIDS or pre-AIDS actually represent responses to disorganised self-antigens arising from endogenous processes, most notably Graft versus Host (GVH) reactions (see below), rather than against the presumed pathogen - HIV is discussed.

Conversely, certain antibodies - e.g. rheumatoid factor - characteristic of certain autoimmune diseases, also occur in infectious diseases, especially in tuberculosis.

It is the purpose of this chapter to give a brief account of the basics of immunology so that some of the wider issues being discussed can be better understood.

THE DEVELOPMENT AND FUNCTIONS OF THE LYMPHOID CELL-LINES

B-cells are concerned with antibody production (originally known as the humoral system) and the T-cells are those concerned with the cellular aspects of the immune system.

In brief, the B-cells develop mainly in the bone marrow-hence 'B' - and the T-cells develop mainly in the thymus-hence 'T'. The stem cells are apparently pluripotential and initially capable of development into all types of blood cell. Cells destined to grow to be lymphocytes first become restricted, then more committed, after which they reach the resting stage in readiness for action when needed.

B-LYMPHOCYTES

These make up about 25% of circulating lymphocytes and their main function is to synthesise and secrete antibodies, which are globular glycoproteins (hence immunoglobulins) found in the blood plasma. On presentation of antigen to the B-cell receptor either directly or after partial digestion within a presenting cell such as a macrophage, and with some 'help' from the CD-4 cells (see below) the B-cells turn into antibody-producing plasma cells producing antibody specific to the invading antigen. The antigen and specific antibody combine to form a complex which with the assistance of complement (see below), becomes engulfed and eliminated by other blood cells..

After the successful removal of the antigen the increased B-cell population reverts to its original level.

The specific antibodies just mentioned are made available due the immunological system's possession of millions of antibodies from which the 'best fit' for the antigen can be selected (Isenberg and Morrow 1995).

THE MAJOR HISTOCOMPATIBILITY COMPLEX (MHC)

The MHC is a group of genes, located on the short arm of chromosome 6, that produce surface markers important both in immune regulation and responses, as just discussed, and in organ transplantation. The HLA antigens are distributed throughout the body and it is through this system that cells can be classified as self or non-self. It is thus the basic means by which appropriate responses can be made to each of these types of antigens i.e. to tolerate self antigens and to attack and remove alien ones.

The human leukocyte antigens became a subject for intense research in the nineteen fifties after the discovery of the occurrence of antibodies to them in sera from blood transfusion recipients and multiparous women. Since then three classes of MHC - I, II and III - products have been described and their structures and functions determined. Only Classes I and II need concern us here.

In the MHC Class I region three molecules are encoded called HLA-A, HLA-B and HLA-C, and are found on most nucleated cells to varying degrees whilst only remnants are found on the red blood cells. The MHC Class II products DW, DR, DQ and DP are found on particular immuno-competent cells including B-lymphocytes, activated T-lymphocytes, dendritic cells and some epithelial cells.

T-LYMPHOCYTES AND THE TRIMOLECULAR COMPLEX

Whereas B-lymphocytes recognise intact extra-cellular antigens, T-lymphocytes recognise intra-cellular ones presented at the surface of body cells. In addition, T-cells only recognise antigen presented in the presence of the self antigens (MHC/HLA components) of the host. Of the two main types of T-cell, the CD-8 cytotoxic/suppressor ones recognise fragments associated with MHC Class I and the other, the CD-4 - the helper - ones recognise those presented with MHC Class II.

The T-cells of both sorts recognise the shape of the antigen fragment/MHC arrangement and the combination of this with the T-cell Receptor (TCR) is known as the trimolecular complex (Fig. 6.1).

When viruses are being assembled within an infected cell, fragments of them become associated with Class I MHC molecules and these complexes are transferred to the surface of the cell to be introduced to the CD-8 cells for killing and elimination.

Fig. 6.1 The Trimolecular Complex

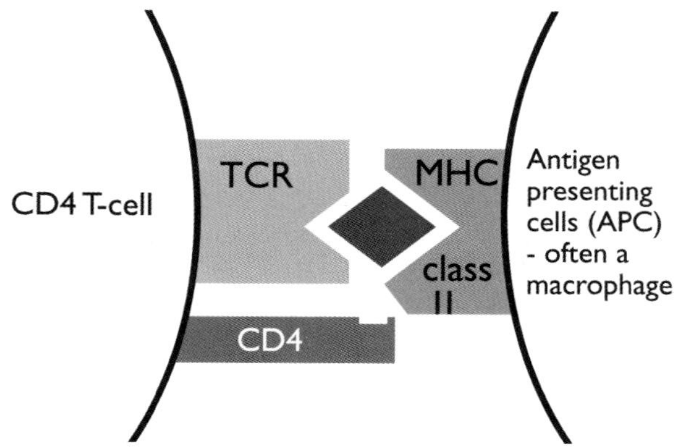

Fig. 6.1 Antigen presentation to a CD-4 cell. CD-4 cells are regarded as critical in AIDS patients in which they occur in low numbers. They are used as one of the monitors for assessing the course the disease is taking. (Chapter Eight)

A similar *modus operandi* for antigen-fragment presentation obtains with CD-4 cells except that the antigen presenting cells (APCs) e.g. macrophages, are more specialised. On recognition of the MHC-antigen complexes on the APC the CD-4 cells release chemicals (cytokines) which are able to activate the APC to destroy the intracellular viruses.

Moreover, on recognition of antigen-MHCs on B-cells, the CD-4 cells can release activating cytokines which 'help' the B-cells to divide and produce appropriate specific antibodies. Other cells exhibiting antigen/MHC complexes recognisable by the CD-4 cells may also be activated by the release of cytokines.

TISSUE TYPING

There are two main techniques for the determination of the tissue type of an individual, and the choice of which is to be employed depends upon the type of HLA antigen to be detected. One technique involves detection of cytotoxicity in response to the homologous antibody of the HLA antigen, and the other, which is more complicated to perform, involves a cell-mediated assay.

In the cytotoxicity assay, an individual's lymphocytes are added to a panel of antisera that are coated in microtitration wells, and after incubation and the addition of complement and a stain, the wells are examined under the microscope. Cytolysis, which indicates homology between the particular antibody and the lymphocytes under investigation, is indicated by the entry of the stain into the dead cells. HLA-A, B and C can be detected in this way. Tests for HLA-DR and DQ need to be carried out on the individual's B-cells when this technique is employed.

Another sort of test involves viable lymphocytes in what are called mixed-lymphocyte tests (MCTs). In these, the lymphocytes under investigation are mixed with a panel of lymphocytes of known constitution and then tested for their proliferation. This is tested by the incorporation of radio-labelled thymidine - if there is uptake, the lymphocytes are not of the same type as the test ones.

The most important application is in the transplantation field, where efforts are concentrated on finding organs that provide as close a match as possible between donor and recipient. The main difficulty in achieving successful therapeutic transplantations such as bone marrow, kidney, liver and heart is the recipient's immunological response to the allograft (graft from a non-identical person) which may result in its rejection. The reaction is the result of the host response to incompatible HLAs in the graft. In addition, such HLA testing may be a useful adjunct in diagnosis of disease, and in paternity testing.

THE COMPLEMENT SYSTEM

The complement system also encoded on chromosome 6 (Class III products) consists of a series of enzymes which interact in various complicated ways within the immune system. It is an important mediator in cell lysis; in inflammatory reactions; in the removal of antigen/antibody complexes and in aiding the activation of macrophages to destroy unwanted foreign substances (for detailed information on the system see Sheehan 1997).

Its importance in the present context lies in the fixation of complement as a laboratory procedure in tissue typing (see above), in the identification of unknown antigens and antibodies in the diagnosis of infection, and in the detection of complement levels in patients with immune disorders.

SUPERANTIGENS

The production by bacteria of toxins capable of causing considerable damage has been known for a very long time. Some of the best known of these are the staphylococcal enterotoxins, toxic shock and scalded skin syndrome toxins. Other bacteria capable of producing toxins now referred to as superantigens include streptococci and *Mycoplasma arthritidis*. The various manifestations of these substances include pathological skin infiltration, inflammation, lymphadenopathy and diarrhoea, and these are caused by a massive T-cell proliferation.

It is now understood that these antigens can by-pass the normal MHC restrictions and are capable of activating up to ten per cent of the mouse cell repertoire, whereas normal reactions activate only a fraction of one per cent (Hoffman 1990; see also Marrack and Kappler 1990). The possible involvement of superantigens in the aetiology of AIDS has been discussed (Dalgleish 1992) and studied extensively in the case of RA based on the *M.arthritidis* model (Cole 1991, Cole *et al* 2000).

THE HLA-B27 CONNECTION WITH THE SPONDYLOARTHROPATHIES

One of the most celebrated unambiguous discoveries in immunopathology, made simultaneously in two different laboratories, is that of the association between HLA-B27 and ankylosing spondylitis (AS). Some 90 to 96% of AS patients are positive for HLA-B27 compared with the 8% that occurs in the general population (Caffrey and James1973, Schlosstein *et al* 1973).

In an interesting historical account, James (1983) explained how much chance happenings had led to the discovery of the HLA disease association and this is not uncommon in scientific research. A related chance happening was concerned in the next stage in the HLA-B27 story - an event that effectively constituted a big human experiment that was carried out by accident.

This involved an epidemic of bacillary dysentery that occurred on an American ship and which was followed by an outbreak of Reiter's Syndrome (a triad of arthritis, conjunctivitis and urethritis). As the author (Noer 1966) put it, chance events conspired with the environment of the crew to produce a setting not unlike a carefully designed scientific experiment. The vessel was already at sea when the outbreak of Shigellosis (dysentery) occurred.

The infection was apparently acquired at a picnic ashore where a considerable amount of food was handled by two cooks who had already become infected. Out of the crew of 1276, 602 suffered from dysentery and of these, ten acquired Reiter's Syndrome, most within two weeks. This in fact amounted to a small epidemic and Noer considered that it could be regarded as a sequel to bacillary dysentery. Moreover, he concluded that some factor common to the ten was somehow causative or at least a triggering mechanism.

Some ten years after Noer's publication and actually thirteen years after the ship epidemic, during which time the connection between AS, HLA-B27 and Reiter's Syndrome had been discovered (Aho *et al* 1974), Colin and Fries (1976) performed a follow-up study on the five of Noer's Reiter's Syndrome patients who could be traced. Their findings were that one of the five cases had minimal disease, was symptom-less and was HLA-B27 negative, whereas the other four had continuous active disease and were all HLA-B27 positive. Thus a definite link between bacteria, tissue type (in this case *Shigella*, HLA-B27), and disease became established.

Although this problem is discussed further in Chapter Nine there are two points worth mentioning at this stage. One is that HLA-B27 positivity is not a genetic defect *per se* but is a marker for ankylosing spondylitis when it fits in with the other characteristics of the disorder - and since only a relatively small number of HLA-B27 positive persons suffer from the disease, there must be other factor(s) involved in those that do. Secondly, it is suggested in later chapters that the AIDS epidemic has features that suggest the life-styles of the 'at risk' groups also constitute settings somewhat like carefully designed scientific experiments - in this case on a world wide scale (Chapters Eight and Nine).

GRAFT VERSUS HOST REACTIONS IN CHIMERAS

The possibility of graft rejection in transplantation has already been mentioned, and in this section the converse of this *i.e.* the reaction of the graft material (transplant) against its host will be considered. In this situation two or more genetically distinct types of cell exist in the body, and the human or animal housing them is called a chimera. According to the circumstances the situation may be tolerated and harmless, or may give rise to serious disease known as graft versus host disease (GVHD).

When the situation causes disease the name of allo-immune disease can reasonably be applied and it is this concept of immunological disease that is the basis of the NGE aetiology that I have already proposed (Pease 1965). The discovery of the HLA system suggests that the infective DNA conveyed by the bacterial vector codes for proteins relating to the definition of self (Burnet's integrity of the body) as compared with those concerned with growth control mechanisms already discussed in Chapter Four with respect to plant cancer and in the next chapter which concerns human cancers.

The similarities between GVHD and such diseases *e.g.* Sjogren's syndrome (SS), scleroderma and primary biliary cirrhosis (PBC) have been recognised for many years. More recently the possibility that these disorders, which affect women predominantly, may be associated with microchimerism that occurs during pregnancy is discussed in Chapter Eight.

The very marked clinical resemblance between AIDS and GVHD was recognised well before the discovery of HIV, which diverted attention from this approach for many years. The GVHD basis for the aetiology of AIDS in terms of the NGE theory is discussed in Chapter Nine.

BENIGN CHIMERISM

One of the natural mechanisms by which this condition occurs is in the case of dizygotic (non-identical twins). One of the first examples of this to be recognised was that of a healthy young blood donor who was found to have 61% group A erythrocytes and 39% of group 0. The latter were found to be those that 'really' belonged to her twin brother who had died in infancy. The two ova were different but the twins shared a common placenta so that their blood cells and their precursors circulated freely from one to the other (Burnet 1962). Such cases are now well recognised, as is the fact that where two sorts of cells are circulating in this way, the individuals fail to develop the antibodies (isoagglutinins) normally associated with the blood groups to which they belong.

Similar cases have been known in cattle for a very long time and 'wrong' cells are found to exist comfortably not only in non-identical calves but also semi-fraternal ones (as in cases of super-fecundation), by virtue of having an inter-connected circulatory system. This type of evidence leads to the conclusion that foreign antigens may be tolerated by an animal that has been exposed to them in the embryonic condition and this has been claimed to provide the main mechanism of tolerance of the animal's own antigenic constituents.

Support for this notion was provided experimentally by prenatal injection of suitable animals. It was shown that mice could be made tolerant of otherwise unacceptable skin grafts by a process of desensitisation in the embryonic stage. The essential features of such sensitisation, either to blood antigens of a type normally destroyed by the subject's constitutional antibodies, or to skin grafts from another individual, that would normally he rejected, are that it should take place in the embryonic stage, and that the desensitising antigens, if the effect is to last, should be living cells capable of establishing themselves, and apparently of reproducing indefinitely.

In simple terms, two stocks of mice are envisaged, one W (White) and the other B (Black), both being inbred to the extent that they are capable of accepting grafts from mice from the same stock but not from the other. If embryo spleen or kidney cells are taken from black mouse embryos and injected into white mouse ones of the same age (or just after birth) the white mouse embryos, all things being equal, will be born naturally and mature apparently normally. The difference from the standard white stock mice is that these become capable by the age of 6-8 weeks of accepting skin grafts from black stock mice. The fact that the black skin graft is still foreign, even though it is tolerated, is demonstrable by the fact that the injection of cells from the spleen or lymph nodes from a normal adult white mouse will cause graft rejection.

GRAFT VERSUS HOST DISEASE - DISEASE-CAUSING CHIMERISM

GVHD is easily demonstrated in mice. The basis of this demonstration is the same as that used for the induction of tolerance but in this case instead of injecting the newborn white mice with black mice embryonic cells, they are injected with cells from adult black mouse spleens. In this case, although the skin graft is tolerated, the graft i.e. the adult foreign cells, will not tolerate the host and GVHD develops.

Table 6.1 Tissue Reactions between Mice W and B (After Burnet 1962)

Donor	Type of Transfer	Recipient W	Recipient B	Recipient WB
W Adult	Skin Graft to Adult	+	-	+
B Adult		-	+	+
WB Adult		-	-	+
W Adult	Spleen to Newborn	n/r	GVHD	GVHD
B Adult		GVHD	n/r	GVHD
WB Adult		n/r	n/r	n/r
W Embryo	Spleen or Kidney to Newborn	n/r	T	n/r
B Embryo		T	T	n/r
WB Embryo		T	T	n/r

+ Graft accepted; - Graft rejected; n/r no reaction; T-Graft tolerated

In theory, W and B represent two pure lines of mouse having distinct differences in their tissue antigens and carrying different gene alleles (variant forms of a gene) at the mouse histocompatability locus H-2. In these experiments three types of mice are involved i.e. W, B and the hybrid F1 (first filial generation).

The production of GVHD requires that the lymphoid donor cells be tolerated for an adequate amount of time in which to become established. If adult spleen cells from either strain are injected into the other one the injected cells do not, of course, survive.

In summary, for W cells, for instance, to survive in B, the latter recipient must be either a) under 24 hr old, b) irradiated sufficiently for destruction of its own lymphoid tissue or c) a hybrid F1 with B as a parent. GVHD in human immunopathologies is discussed further in Chapter Nine.

HETEROPHILE ANTIBODIES

Antibodies elicited by antigen from one source may be capable of reacting with a structurally similar one from a genetically unrelated other source, and these are known as heterophile antibodies. These cross reactions occur between unrelated microorganisms and between microorganisms and animal tissues. In the former case the cross-reactivity may be an aid to diagnosis, the classic example being the diagnosis of typhus fever in the Weil-Felix reaction. The latter has been suggested as being responsible for some manifestations of autoimmunity, and this is discussed in Chapter Nine.

THE WEIL-FELIX REACTION

The rickettsiae are small bacteria that are obligate intracellular parasites and which cause a variety of severe diseases. They occur under natural conditions in the gut of blood-sucking arthropods e.g. lice, fleas, mites and ticks, and when transmitted to man some cause typhus and related diseases. The bacteria are difficult and time consuming to grow and dangerous to handle, but diagnosis has been made easy because of the cross-reactivity that exists between the rickettsiae and certain strains of *Proteus*, an unrelated bacterium which is safe and easy to handle in the laboratory.

The reaction, first described by Weil and Felix, is very simple to carry out and of great practical importance in the diagnosis of rickettsial infections. In epidemic typhus the titre of agglutinins for *Proteus* OX 19 has usually reached a figure of 200 after one week of illness and a peak of 1000-5000 is reached at the end of the second week. The agglutinins tend to disappear a few months after recovery and thus a positive Weil-Felix reaction is a useful indication of recent infection. (Table 6.2)

Table 6.2 Weil-Felix Tests

Disease	Vectors	Proteus Strains		
		OX19	OX2	OXK
Rocky Mounted Spotted Fever	Tick-borne	+++	++	-
Fièvre Boutonneuse		++	++	-
South African Tick Bite Fever		++	++	-
Murine Typhus	Flea-borne	+++	+	-
Tsutsugamushi Fever	Mite-borne	-	-	+++

The results of the Weil-Felix test should be interpreted strictly in relation to the clinical findings, for a positive reaction is occasionally observed in other diseases such as undulant fever, malaria, infectious mononucleosis and tuberculosis.

MOLECULAR MIMICRY AND RHEUMATIC FEVER

In RF acute symptoms of swollen and painful joints, which accounted for the name of the condition, usually subsided after a time, but involvement of the heart, which often occurred, could be very serious and could lead to death or chronic heart disease. The condition is almost always initiated by an infection with Group A streptococci (*Streptococcus pyogenes*, the type that commonly affects humans causing sore-throat or pharyngitis) which may belong to any of the various M types within the group.

Anti-heart antibodies were reported to occur in the sera of patients with RF and it was found that these antibodies reacted with Group A streptococci; both types of sera were found to cross-react with heart and skeletal muscle. The streptococcal antigens N-acetyl-glucosamine, M protein and cardiac myosin appear to be involved in the cross-reactivity. The interpretation of these observations by some was that the antibody produced to combat the streptococcus takes part in a sensitivity reaction involving the heart and small blood vessels of the patient.

The idea of this so-called molecular mimicry that arose from these sixties studies on Group A streptococci and RF has become firmly entrenched in the philosophy of diseases of immunopathology, either as a cause *per se* or an exacerbating factor, being involved not only in RF but in diseases of immunopathology in general (see Cunningham 2000, 2003 for streptococcal references). The subject of molecular mimicry is discussed further in Chapters Eight and Nine.

SUMMARY

Some of the basics of immunology needed to understand the nature of the disorders under investigation are presented and some of the techniques and approaches for their investigation are explained. The HLA system and its connection with particular diseases is described. Other areas touched upon are Graft versus Host Disease (GVHD), superantigens and molecular mimicry.

REFERENCES

Aho, K., Ahvonen, A., Lassus, A *et al* (1974) HLA-1327 in Reactive Arthritis
Arthritis and Rheumatism <u>17</u> 521-526

Brostoff, J. Scadding, G.K. Male, D.M. *et al* (1991)
Clinical Immunology Gower Medical Publishing, London, New York

Burnet, M. (1962) The Integrity of the Body
Harvard University Press London: Oxford University Press

Caffrey, M.F.P. and James, D.C.0 (1973) Human lymphocyte antigen in ankylosing spondylitis
Nature <u>242</u> 121

Cole, B. C. (1991) The immunobiology of Mycoplasma arthritidis and its superantigen MAM. Curr. *Top. Microbial. Immunol.* 174 107-119

Cole, B.C., Mu, H-H. and Sawitzke, A.D. (2000) The mycoplasma superantigen MAM: Role in arthritis and immune-mediated disease
Int.J Med Microbiol 290 489-490

Colin, A. and Fries, J.F. (1976) An 'Experimental 'Epidemic of Reiter's Syndrome Revisited. Follow up on Genetic and Environmental Factors
Ann.Int. Med. 84 564-556

Cunningham, M.W. (2000) Pathogenesis of Group A Streptococcal Infections
Clinical Microbiology Reviews July 470-511

Cunningham M. W. (2003) Autoimmunity and molecular mimicry in the pathogenesis of post-streptococcal heart disease
Front Riosci 8 533-543

Hoffman, M. (1990) 'Superantigens' may shed light on immune puzzle
Science 248 685-686

Dalgleish, A.G. (1992) The pathogenesis of AIDS: classical and alternative views
Journal of the Royal College of Physicians of London 26 152-158

Isenberg, D. and Morrow, J. (1995) Friendly Fire: Explaining Autoimmune Disease
Oxford University Press

James, D.C.O. (1983) HLA-B27 in Clinical Medicine - Historical Reflections on the Discovery of the Disease Association
British J. of Rheumatology 22 (Suppl 2) 20-24

Marrack, P. and Kappler J. (1990) The Staphylococcal Enterotoxins and their relatives
Science 248 705-711

Noer, H (1966) An 'Experimental' Epidemic of Reiter's Syndrome
J.A.M.A. 197 117-122

Schlosstein, L., Terasaki, P.I., Bluestone, R. et al (1973) High association of HLA antigen W27 with ankylosing spondylitis
New.Eng.J.Med 288 704-706

Sheehan, C (1997) Clinical immunology: Principles and Laboratory Diagnosis 2nd Ed Lippincott Williams and Wilkins

Thomas, L (1971) Adaptive aspects of inflammation. in Immunopathology of inflammation (ed 5.K. Forsher and J.C. Houck) Amsterdam: Excerpta Medica.
As quoted by Taylor, F.J.R. in The Cell as Habitat. The Royal Society London 1979.

CHAPTER SEVEN

THE MALIGNANCIES

'There is no inevitability of a smooth, regular progress in scientific research and many things, so it seems, have to be discovered and rediscovered several times until they find the right ambience, the correct context of contemporary thought they need before they can be understood and accepted'.

K.A. Bisset (1962)

'The great importance which a knowledge of botany possesses for the pathologist lies in this, that it enables him to discover in all these processes the existence of an inward correspondence in the whole series of vital phenomena, and to show how the lowest formations may serve to explain the history of the most perfect and complex parts'.

R. Virchow (1871)

'Let us note to begin with that the cancers of plants are in many respects strikingly similar to those in animals. They can be initiated by many of the same kinds of agents; the transformed cells grow without control by the host plant; they reproduce true to the tumour type and they lack the structure and functions of normal cells. In short, they show the essential biological characteristics of malignant animal cells'.

A. C. Braun (1965)

'The ground rules (of DNA replication and proliferation) are of very old evolutionary origin, conserved and shared by different cell types and tissues'.

M. Greaves (1997)

INTRODUCTION 87

THE ORIGIN AND CLONAL EVOLUTION OF HUMAN CANCERS 88

THE LEUKAEMIAS 89

THE STEPS IN THE PROGRESSION TO MALIGNANCY IN PLANTS 91

THE ROLE OF HORMONES IN PLANT CANCER 92

continued overleaf

contents continued

THE ROLE OF NEO-VASCULARIZATION (ANGIOGENESIS) IN PLANT AND HUMAN CANCER 92

MUTATIONS, MUTATIONS, MUTATIONS! 94

HERITABLE CANCERS AND TUMOUR SUPPRESSOR GENES 95

LEUKAEMIAS ORIGINATING *IN UTERO* 96

INFECTION AND/OR IRRADIATION IN CHILDHOOD LEUKAEMIAS 97

SOLID TUMOURS AS LATER STAGES IN CANCER PROGRESSION 99

RSV/*SRC* AS A MODEL FOR HUMAN CANCER 101

BACTERIA AS ALTERNATIVE VECTORS OF ALIEN GROWTH-CONTROLLING DNA 101

THE HUMAN BACTERIAL ENDOPARASITE 102

SUMMARY 105

INTRODUCTION

Cancer is a disorder of multicellular creatures and occurs as a result of a cell (or cells) within the organisation (plant, animal or human) somehow gaining a growth advantage over the co-existing cells, which allows it to proliferate more freely and to proceed to further increasingly unfettered multiplication by a step by step process and eventually to invasion of other parts of the body where a suitable transport (vascular) system exists.

In many cases the cells are able to grow in the laboratory on simple media in the absence of the host, thus achieving a sort of immortality and living for many years after the death of the original host - human, animal or plant. Biology by definition involves the study of life in all its forms, and in the present context most significantly the study of the biological phenomenon of the balance between birth, growth (maturation) and decay (death), and from this viewpoint these processes are essentially the same in animals, humans and plants.

It is the thinking in this chapter that the most obvious differences between plants and animals i.e. the possession of specialised organs in animals, that are simplified or non-existent in plants, and the fact that plants have rigid cell-walls, are the ones that make the study of their cancers such a good model for the animal and human ones. Whilst these characteristics do not in any way detract from the philosophy of the essential sameness of the cancer process in multicellular organisms, the ease of handling plant material helps to elucidate various factors such as the impact of hormones in the steps towards malignancy, which can then be and applied to the much more highly complex human and animal systems.

Currently the retrovirus *onc/gene* model discussed in chapter five is regarded as an aberration of nature, which may supply some pointer to cancer in humans, but nothing more. Furthermore the plant cancer model (Chapter Four) has escaped the notice of most current cancer investigators as a model for human cancer - its exploitation for the production of genetically engineered crops has overshadowed this. The point that seems to have been missed is that both models show that transfers of alien DNA from one individual to another can cause cancer. Both are mechanisms of natural genetic engineering and it seems inconceivable that such mechanisms do not occur in humans.

In fact one school of thought has long considered that the association of *Agrobacterium*-like bacteria with human cancers might indicate that human and plant cancers could share a common aetiology. This notion received sufficient credibility to engender a meeting on the subject by the New York Academy of Sciences in November 1969 when the subject was debated once more and the subsequent discovery of the *modus operandi* of plant cancer added even more credibility to the idea (Pease 1990).

Research on human cancer today, in the absence of a recognised general cause, is necessarily concentrated on the later stages of the disease. These are mainly directed towards the understanding of cellular control mechanisms and how these processes can go wrong in ways that can cause cancer and also to the extension of the study of chromosome aberrations with the idea of improving determinations of prognoses and the choice of therapy for the treatment of patients. The role of genomic instability and its place in tumour development still remain a matter of controversy.

In this chapter I am suggesting a return to the setting that existed before the wrong turning to retrovirology was taken in 1970 and to re-examine the bacterial vector one, as a cause of at least some human cancers, whilst taking into account the more recent discoveries that have been made in the various stages in the development of these cancers.

THE ORIGIN AND CLONAL EVOLUTION OF HUMAN CANCERS

Nowell (1976), one of the co-discoverers of the Philadelphia (Ph) chromosome phenomenon in 1960, proposed a model of tumour evolution which in general terms in still valid today. This is diagrammatically represented in Fig 7.1. He suggested, basing his evidence on cytogenetic and biochemical studies that the process begins with an induced change in a previously normal cell (N), which then becomes neoplastic and somehow gains a growth advantage over the adjacent normal cells. Proliferation of this clone (descendents from the original neoplastic cell) takes place either immediately or after a rest period.

Fig. 7.1 Model of Clonal Evolution in Neoplasia (After Nowell 1976)

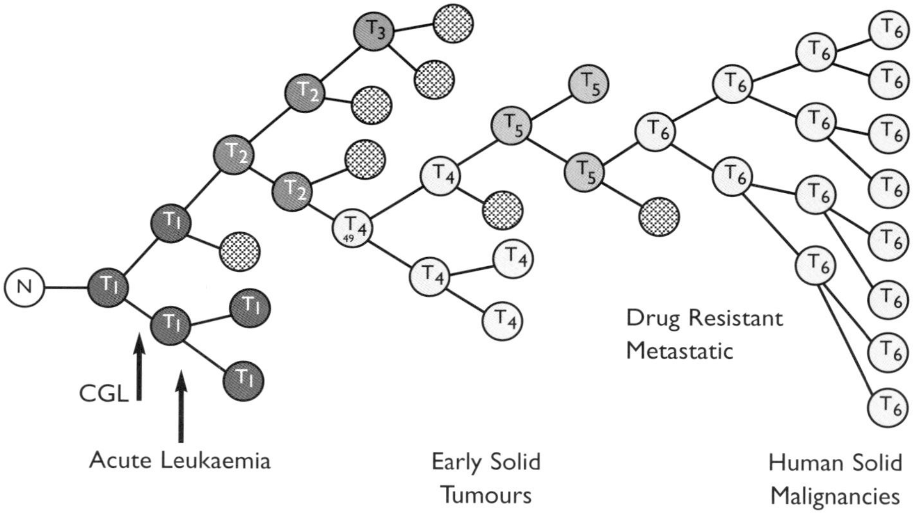

Fig. 7.1. Model of clonal evolution in neoplasia. Carcinogen-induced change in progenitor normal cell (N) produces a diploid tumour cell (T1, 46 chromosomes) with growth advantage permitting clonal expansion to begin. Genetic instability of T-cells leads to production of variants (illustrated by changes in chromosome number (T2 to T6). Most variants die, due to metabolic or immunologic disadvantage (hatched circles); occasionally one has an additional selective advantage (for example, 12, 47 chromosomes), and its progeny become the predominant subpopulation until an even more favourable variant appears (for example, T4). The stepwise sequence in each tumour differs, (being partially determined by environmental pressures on selection) and results in a different, aneuploid karyotype in each fully developed malignancy (T.6). Biological characteristics of tumour progression (for example, morphological and metabolic loss of differentiation, invasion and metastasis, resistance to therapy) parallel the stages of genetic evolution. Human tumours with minimal chromosome change (diploid acute leukaemia, chronic granulocytic leukaemia) are considered to be early in clonal evolution; human solid cancers, typically highly aneuploid, are viewed as late in the developmental process.
Suggested chromosome numbers in this model T2, 47 - T3, 48 -T4,49 - T5, 98 and T6, 97.
CGL =Chronic Granulocytic Leukaemia in which the Philadelphia chromosome occurs (Fig. 7.2)

Subsequently, mutations take place in the neoplastic clone as a result of genetic instability and although many of these are eliminated because they are disadvantaged in some way, occasionally one mutation gives the cell an advantage in growth potential, and this proliferates and becomes the precursor of a new predominant sub-population of cells. This essentially evolutionary process continues, and the developing cells become more and more abnormal both genetically and biologically. Although some similarities become common in tumour cells, other characteristics are acquired in response to local environmental conditions and give rise to variant sub-lines and eventually the tumour becomes unique in its karyotype, antigenic properties and bizarre metabolic characteristics. At this stage of full malignancy the potential for variation still persists, making possible the emergence of resistance of the tumour to irradiation and chemotherapy.

The step by step process thus involves the transition from normal cell to benign solid tumour and eventually to malignant solid tumour. In this model the leukaemias are regarded as being early in clonal evolution. The steps are accompanied by chromosome aberrations and less visible mutations in the developing cancer cells- their DNA may have deletions, insertions, duplications, translocations and base substitutions, and although the major aberrations have been recognised as being a diagnostic aid in cancer for over a hundred years there is still no agreement about their exact significance and what causes their development and, except for some specialised cases, the time of their occurrence during the disease process is uncertain. This is discussed further below.

THE LEUKAEMIAS

Nowell regarded the leukaemias as being early in the clonal evolution of cancer, and the classic Ph chromosome is an example of a first step in cancer evolution that is visible at chromosomal level, relatively early in the disease process (Fig. 7.2).

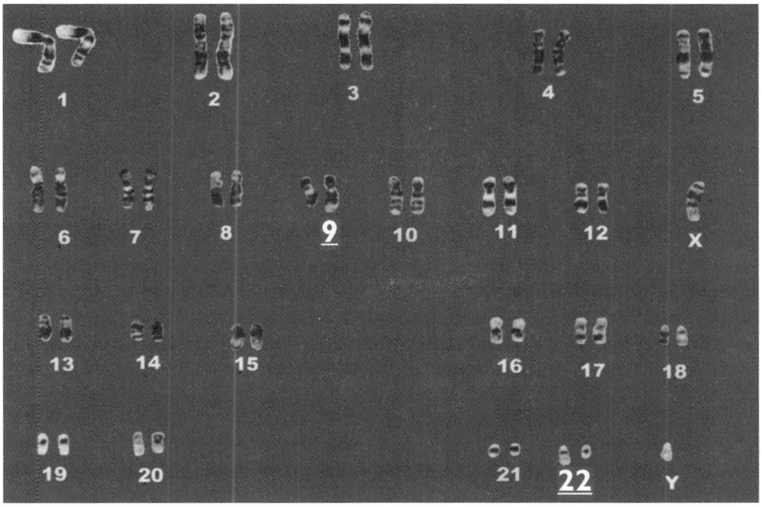

Fig. 7.2. Human somatic cells normally have 46 chromosomes, and chromosome analysis is carried out on cells in the course of cell-division when the chromosomes become separated. Each chromosome can be identified by size, shape and staining properties and a full picture of the chromosomes in a cell obtained. The first specific chromosome aberration in human cancer was observed in patients with chronic myeloid/granulocytic

leukaemia by Nowell and Hungerford in Philadelphia in 1960. The abnormality, which occurs in 85-90% of CML patients, is the reciprocal translocation between chromosomes 9 and 22 which gives rise to a small chromosome 22 i.e. the so-named Philadelphia (Ph) chromosome. There is evidence that the 9-22 hybrid contributes to the progression of the disease, but the basic question of what actually causes the aberration is still not understood. It has often been referred to as the 'first hit' by cancer research workers but the possibility is that it is the result rather than the cause of the beginning of the malignant process. There are some parallels here with the situation that exists in AIDS, where the diagnostic test is for sero-positivity to the p24 antigen has not been explained to the satisfaction of several investigators (Chapter Eight).

The appearance of this translocation between chromosomes 9 and 22 marks what is referred to as the 'first hit' in the progression of CML, which when followed by a 'second hit' causes a relapse into a progressively malignant phase. This process has been admirably illustrated by Greaves (Fig. 7.3).

Fig. 7.3 Clonal Selection and Cellular Phenotypes in Leukaemias (After Greaves 1991)

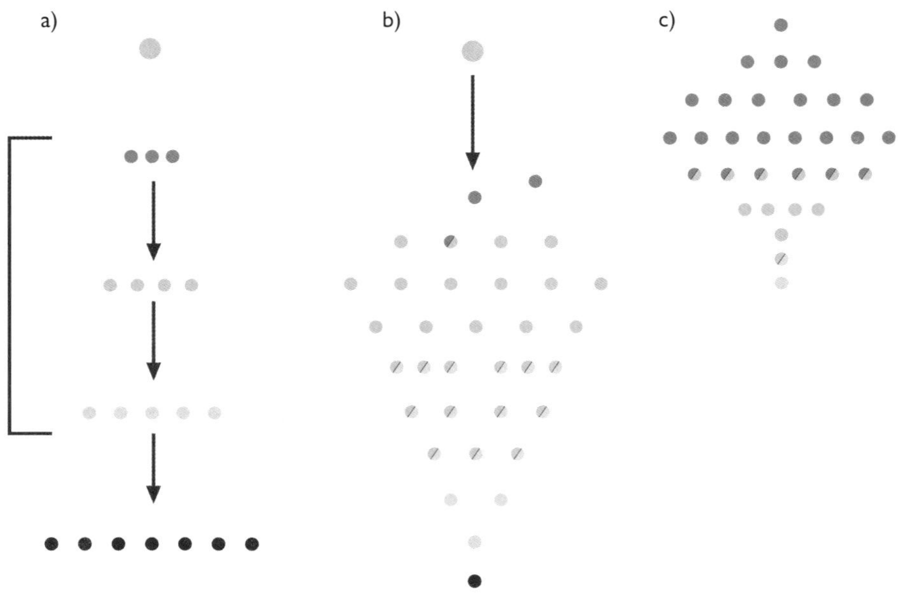

Fig 7.3 a) This shows the normal developmental sequence from stem cells to mature ones b) A leukaemic clone and c) a sub-clone of b in relapse. b and c show an uncoupling of proliferation and differentiation causing abortive maturation and some asynchrony of phenotypes (mixed colour cells) The first genetic transforming event (1) occurs in a primitive stem cell or one of its immediate progeny. The second (2) genetic event occurs in a poorly differentiated cell within the leukaemic clone, which gives it a further selective growth advantage - and perhaps drug resistance - and produces a dominant with even more maturation arrest. Reproduced by permission of Professor Mel Greaves.

The multistep process and clonal nature of human cancers are most readily demonstrated in the blood cancers i.e. the leukaemias, lymphomas and myelomas because a) it is relatively simple to obtain blood and bone marrow samples for the direct examination for chromosome and other abnormalities and b) it is much easier to establish cell-lines from the relevant blood cells than it is from solid tumours.

THE STEPS IN THE PROGRESSION TO MALIGNANCY IN PLANTS

Plant tumours are solid ones, and in a sense provide a model intermediate between the leukaemias and the solid human ones, and since the tumours can be induced and examined at will, the access to this information is infinitely simpler than in either of the others. The nature of plant tumours enables them to be examined very easily in stained sections and this is the technique used by Erwin Smith, by which he demonstrated very elegantly the essential similarity between human and plant cancers. Some of the best illustrations of the progression of normal cells to malignant ones were produced by Smith (1922) from tumours produced in the cortex of a young tobacco plant by inoculating it with his Paris daisy strain *via* a needle prick (Figs. 7.4).

The sections were made from the resulting tumour at the age of three weeks. In fact, the slides were not examined for several years - these things happen in laboratories - but on re-staining and inspection, a 0.5 mm. zone containing cells intermediate in characteristics between the normal cortex cells and the overt tumour cells was apparent.

Fig. 7.4 Steps in the Progression to Malignancy in a Tobacco Plant Tumour Showing Similarities to the Steps to Leukaemia (After Smith 1922 and Braun 1965)

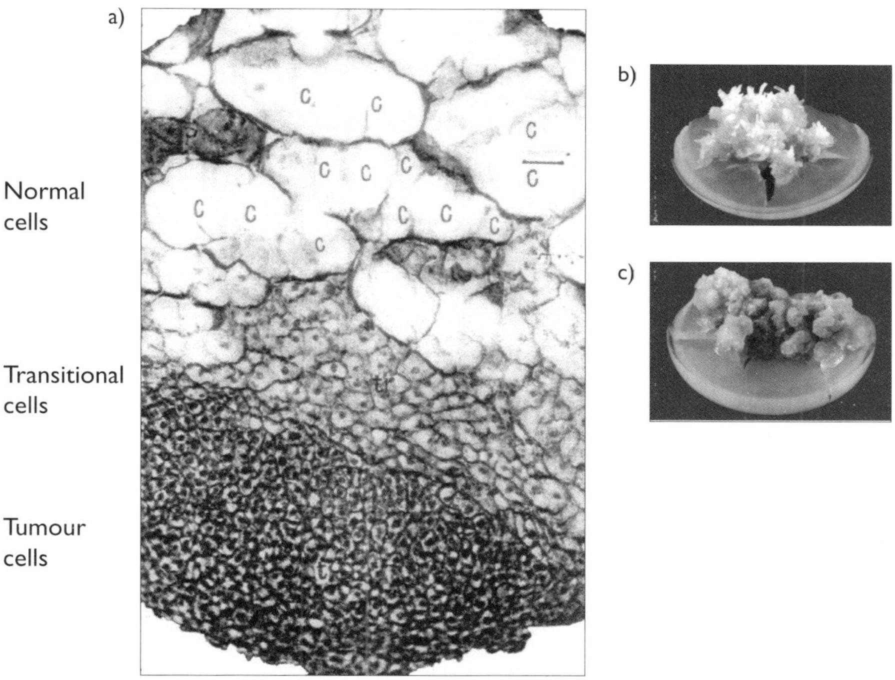

Fig. 7.4 a) This is a section of an A. *tumefaciens*-induced tobacco plant tumour showing the normal, transitional and disorganised tumour cells. b) Growth of intermediate transitional cells cultured on minimal medium. Some differentiation is apparent,. c) Fully autonomous growth on minimal medium equivalent to a relapse in leukaemia.

THE ROLE OF HORMONES IN PLANT CANCER

Early investigators discovered that plant hormones, the auxins that control the growth in size of the cells and the cytokinins and auxins controlling their proliferation are central in establishing abnormal growth.

Mature normal cells do not produce these hormones, but on transformation into tumour cells, by wounding and infection, they become progressively more able to produce these growth factors for themselves, the normal regulatory systems become disorganised and the cells eventually become completely autonomous and grow on minimal medium away from the plant. The steps to malignancy can be demonstrated in culture by varying the plant hormone/growth factor elements in the culture medium (Figs. 7.5) and these parallel the stages shown in the tumour sections.

Hormones play a very large part in human cancer, and cancer endocrinology has been the subject of a vast number of studies for over a century, particularly with the object of providing a cure, especially in breast cancer. Tamoxifen, which is used as an anti-oestrogen, has been particularly effective in this area. Obviously the situation in humans is infinitely more complicated than that obtaining in plants, but the fundamental mechanism of a cell or cells breaking loose from the normal restraints by means of mutations - known to be insertional *via* alien DNA in the plants - is similar.

Fig. 7.5 The Effect of Growth Regulators on the Progression of Normal Plant Cells to Malignancy

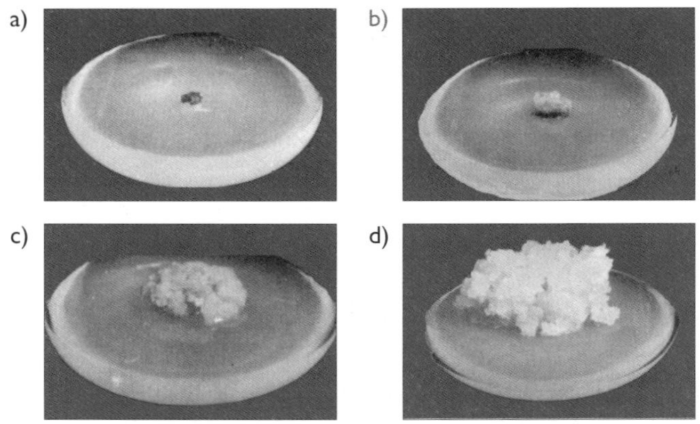

Fig. 7,5 a) These are normal plant cells that can be grown in culture only with the addition of cytokinin, which triggers cell-division and auxin, inositol, aspartic acid, cytodylic and guanylic acids (the building bricks of DNA. b) Weak slow growing tumour cells - these can be made to grow rapidly by the addition to the medium of auxin, glutamine, inositol, aspartic acid, cytodylic and guanylic acids. c) Moderately growing tumour cells - these are able to produce all growth. d) Fast growing growth without additives.

THE ROLE OF NEO-VASCULARIZATION (ANGIOGENESIS) IN PLANT AND HUMAN CANCER

Another characteristic that plant cancer shares with the human disease is the development of neo-vascularization in the progression of the diseases.

One of the most important requirements for tumour progression in humans is the development of a rich supply of blood vessels to foster the tumour with oxygen and various nutrients. This process, which is known as angiogenesis, enables small (1-2mm), relatively harmless tumours to become larger and so bring about a further step towards full malignancy. This procedure is stimulated by the production of growth factors by the tumour cells and by products associated with the tumour cells deprived of oxygen. This is an exploitation of the normal cell mechanism developed for cell preservation such as wound healing (Greaves 2001). Natural proteins called angiostatin and endostatin are currently being investigated as a means of preventing cancer progression, as they were found to do in some strains of mice, in the hope of finding therapies that do not encourage the emergence of resistance in tumour cells.

In plants, tumours likewise achieve the ability to grow beyond a certain size level - they may reach diameters of more than 100 mm - by means of neo-vascularization. The plant tumours induce the formation of an intricate vascular network of water-conducting and assimilate-transporting sieve elements by the over-expression of the T-DNA-encoded vascularization promoting the plant equivalents of the human growth factors, namely auxin and cytokinin. Increases in auxin production as high as 500 times that of control plants and of cytokinin up to 1600 times that of controls have been reported (Ullrich and Aloni 2000).

Recent work has shown that in addition to the well-known roles of auxin and cytokinin, they also trigger a strong emission of ethylene, which is now known to have an important role in tumourigenesis. It has been demonstrated that in crown-galls initiated by *A.tumefaciens*, tumour-induced ethylene causes the development of pathological xylem characterised by the narrowing of the vessels. This impairs water flow to the shoots above the gall and gives priority of the water supply to the tumour over that of the host. Furthermore, crown galls do not regenerate disrupted epidermis and cuticle so that protection against water evaporation is lost, and transpiration is very much increased to the further advantage of the tumour at the expense of the host.

The effects of ethylene on the genesis of tumours have been elegantly demonstrated by Aloni *et al* (1998) who studied the effects of infection by *Agrobacterium tumefaciens* on wild type tomato (*Lycopersicon esculentum* Mill.) as compared with its ethylene-insensitive mutant Never ripe (Nr). In the wild type the ethylene substantially reduced the vessel diameter of the host tissues close to the tumour but had considerably less effect on the Nr mutant. Ethylene promotes the characteristic unorganised callus shape of the gall and this has the effect of increasing the surface area - and thus transpiration - in the wild type but in the case of the mutant the galls have a smoother, more organised surface. Thus whilst the water flow goes preferentially to the tumour on the wild plant, in the mutant the upper parts of the shoots have an uninterrupted water supply and the tumour size is accordingly reduced or even inhibited. (Fig. 7.6).

Fig 7.6 The Effects of Ethylene on the Development of *A. tumefaciens*-induced Tumours

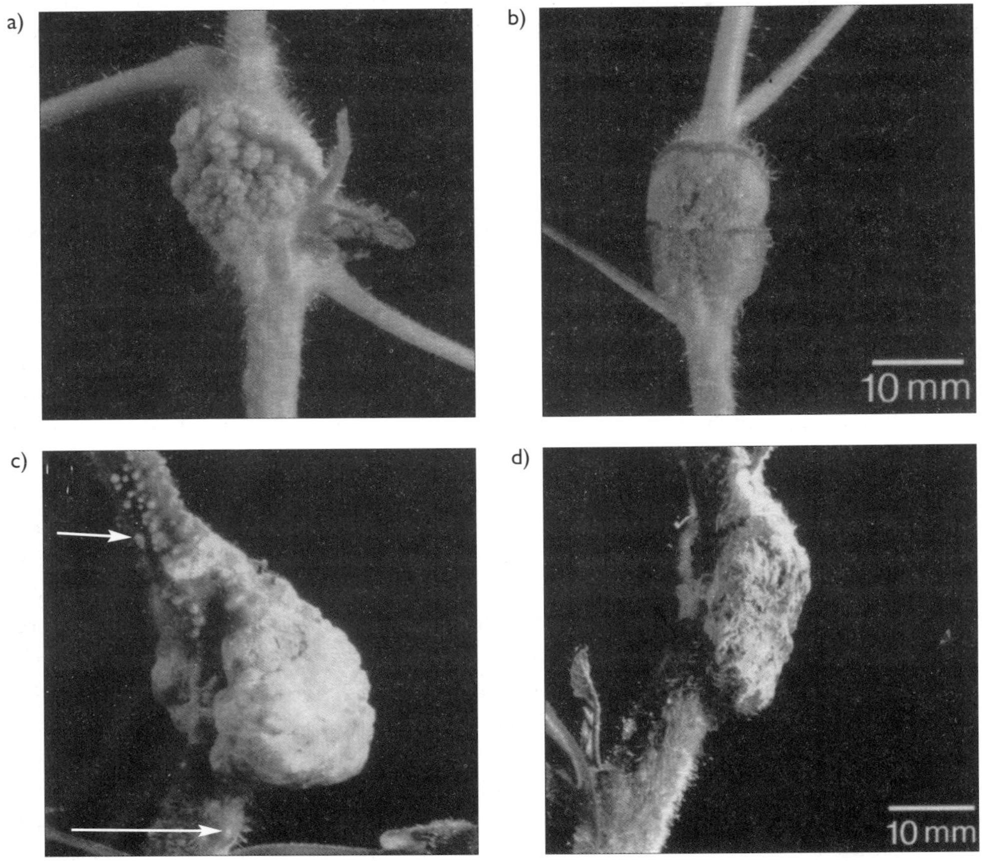

Fig. 7.6. This demonstrates the difference of the effects of *A. tumefaciens* infection on the wild type tomato (a and c) as compared with its ethylene sensitive mutant called Never ripe (*Nr*) (b and d).

a) Front view of a 3-week old tumour developed on a wild type plant showing the showing the typical disorganised callus shape of a young crown gall and the epinastic response both above and below the tumour.

b) Front view of a 3-week old tumour on the *Nr* mutant, characterised by a smooth surface and leaves in the normal position. Note that the lower part of the gall is protected by the epidermis.

c) Side view of the of a 2-month old tumour on a wildtype stem with numerous adventitious roots (arrows) developed both above and below the tumour.

d) Side view of a 2-month old tumour on the *Nr* mutant showing a fibrous hard gall and a stem almost free of adventitious roots.

Illustration kindly provided by Roni Aloni, University of Tel Aviv.

MUTATIONS, MUTATIONS, MUTATIONS!

There is general agreement that human cancer involves a step by step progression from a normal cell to full malignancy but in the case of human cancer as opposed to plant cancer the nature of the cause of the initial transition from normal to neoplastic is unknown.

The significance of the chromosome abnormalities - most cancer cells show striking changes in their karyotypes and these include gains or losses of whole chromosomes, which renders them aneuploid (as opposed to the normal diploid), amplifications and or deletions of genetic material that accompany the progression towards full malignancy is still a matter of debate. Translocations also occur, as already discussed in connection with the Philadelphia chromosome, and in addition vast numbers of mutations occur at the sub-microscopic level during the course of the disease.

Some of these abnormalities are regarded as activators of growth-promoting genes and others as deactivating tumour-suppressing genes and there appears to be general concurrence that the final stages of carcinogenesis result from the accumulation of several such changes or mutations.

The concept of genomic instability - a raised built-in mutation rate - has been under discussion recently, several workers believing that something over and above the mutation rate of normal somatic cells must be switched into action to account for the chaotic state of DNA organisation in the cancer cells.

Some groups believe that this state arises early in the steps to malignancy. Loeb for example, working with mathematical models, introduced the concept of a mutator cell, as a means of accounting for the high rate of mutations in cancer cells compared with the low mutation rates of normal somatic cells. The proposal was that the multiple cancer-associated mutations are the result of mutations already having taken place in the genes that guarantee the fidelity of DNA synthesis or the adequacy of the DNA repair mechanisms, and that this would predispose these cells to the accumulation of additional mutations (Loeb 2001).

Bodmer and his colleagues, (Tomlinson and Bodmer 1999, Tomlinson *et al* 2002) on the other hand, believe that the role of genomic instability has been overestimated, and again by the use of mathematical models have calculated that Loeb and his supporters have actually underestimated the number of cell divisions needed for a the production of a tumour, and their philosophy of cancer development is very much on the side of selective forces being the major prime factor (see also Greaves 2001).

Such speculations on the role of genomic instability in tumour development as well as advances in the understanding of cell control mechanisms have arisen to a large extent from studies on the hereditary cancers, most notably in recent years the colorectal ones, and these will now be discussed.

HERITABLE CANCERS AND TUMOUR SUPPRESSOR GENES

The study of heritable cancer susceptibility genes has provided an insight into genes which, in the simplest terms, control cell proliferation. The most widely known of these genes is the one coding for the p53 (53-kilo Dalton) protein. The short arm of chromosome 17, which harbours this gene, is lost in many human tumours.

P53 was initially discovered as a transformation-associated protein in tissue culture experiments with the small DNA virus SV40, but ten years were to elapse before its role as a tumour suppressor gene was clearly defined. The terms 'guardian of the genome' by Lane and 'cellular gate keeper' by Levine both give an idea of the vital importance of p53 as a guard against undesirable cell proliferation. Currently it is the subject of a big research effort to realise its therapeutic potential (Hupp *et al* 2000).

The pathways involved in its role as a 'decider' of whether cells damaged by various mechanisms e.g. irradiation, chemical carcinogens or infection should be repaired or made to undergo apoptosis are highly complex, and so are the mechanisms devised by rogue cells and/or infective agents to oppose the guardian's protective strategies. Mutations in the p53 gene are present in some fifty per cent of tumours and these mutations are of particular importance when they occur in germ cells. In fact it was a study on germ-line p53 mutations in a familial syndrome of breast cancer, sarcomas and other neoplasms that helped to establish the role of p53 as a tumour suppressor gene.

The Li-Fraumeni syndrome (LFS), a rare heritable cancer susceptibility condition, was first described in 1969. Although it appears in two to four per cent of the population, the probability of the occurrence of various tumours, including sarcomas, leukaemias and lung and breast cancers, by the age of thirty, is fifty per cent as opposed to one percent in the rest of the population. Malkin *et al* (1990) examined five families with the condition and found p53 mutations in all of them.

Vogelstein and his colleagues firmly established the putative role of p53 in laboratory experiments. These (Baker *et al* 1990) involved the transfection and transformation by wild and mutant p53 genes of human colorectal carcinoma lines and showed that the normal p53 gene specifically suppresses the growth of human colorectal carcinoma cells *in vitro* and furthermore that this suppressive activity could be invalidated by a mutation in an *in vivo* derived p53.

Further research on heritable colon cancers, most notably hereditary non-polyposis colon cancer (HNPCC), has led to the identification of other genes, particularly those associated with the repair of DNA, that render cells at risk of further mutations in genes responsible for cellular growth control.

These observations, and many others, too complex to describe in detail, have led to the demonstration of a process similar to that described above of the stepwise nature of plant cancer progression, involving not only histological observations but also the genetic ones in parallel (Kinzler and Vogelstein 1998).

LEUKAEMIAS ORIGINATING *IN UTERO*

The object of this section is to consider how the characteristics of human cancers might be explicable in terms of the *modus operandi* responsible for the alien/allo DNA-inducing cancers in both animal and plant cancers. The question that now needs consideration is how the natural history and clinical course of malignant disease and its correlation with laboratory observations are consistent with the putative alien (from another human) DNA colonisation aetiology. The leukaemias, which are the easiest to follow in these respects, will be considered first.

A general characteristic of leukaemia cells is their ability to survive conditions, particularly shortage of growth factors, which would bring about cell death in normal cells as is the case with plant

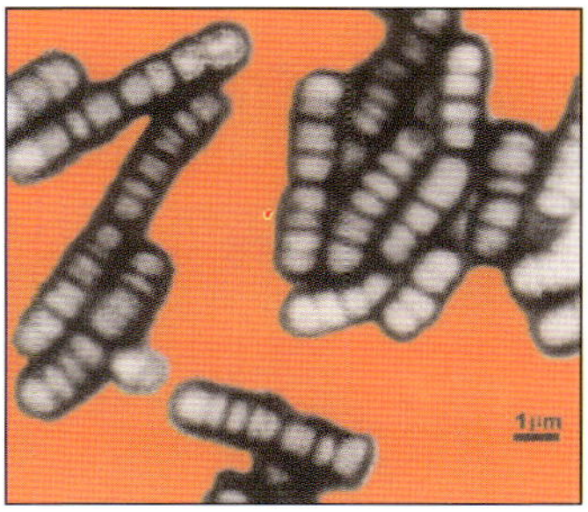

1.1a

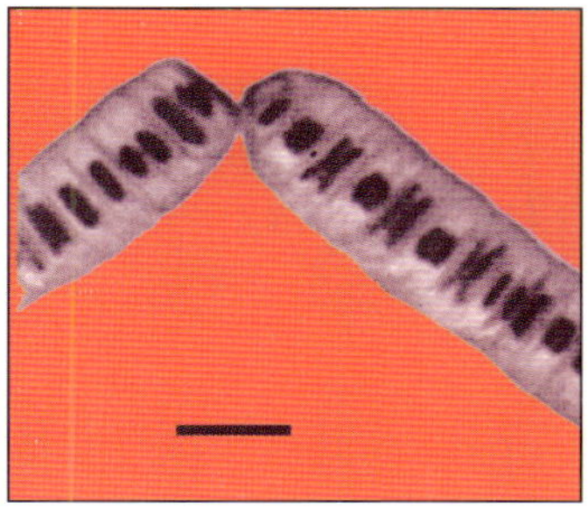

1.1c

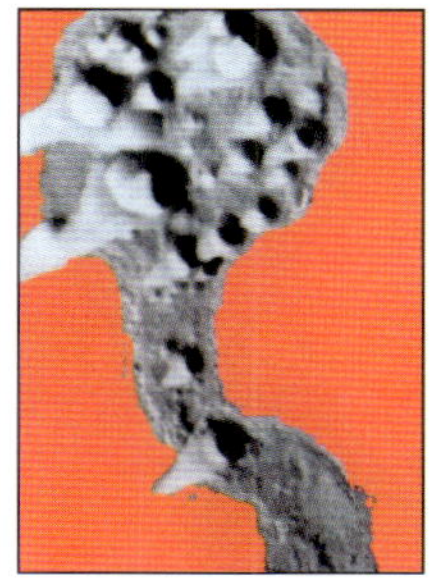

1.3b

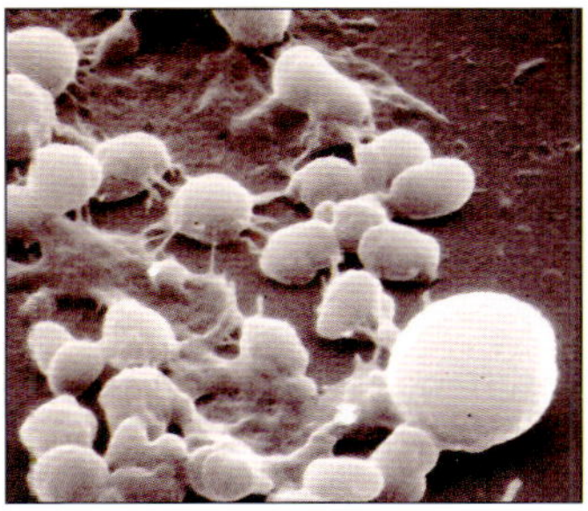

1.4b

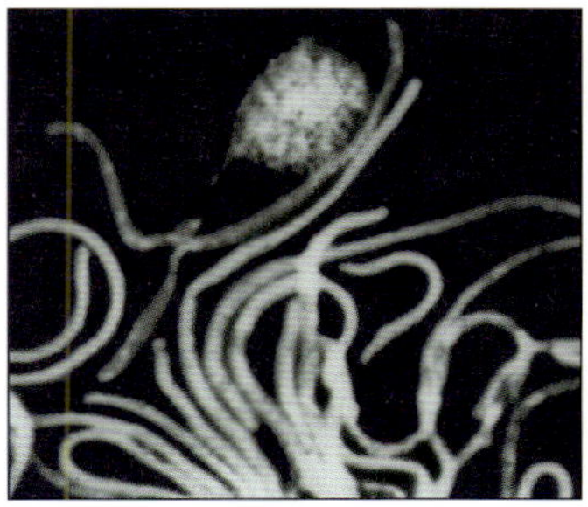

1.2d

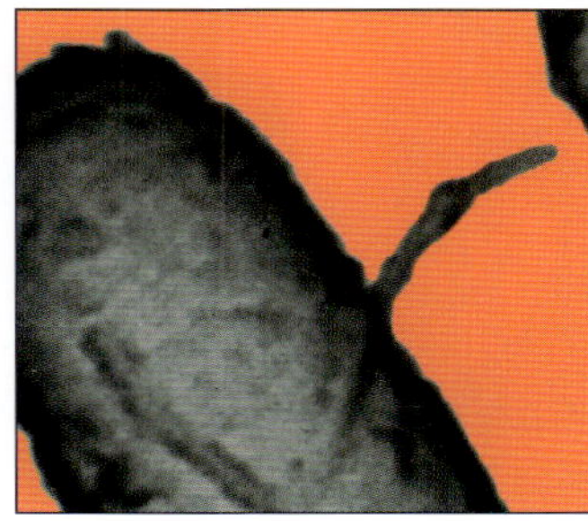

1.5c

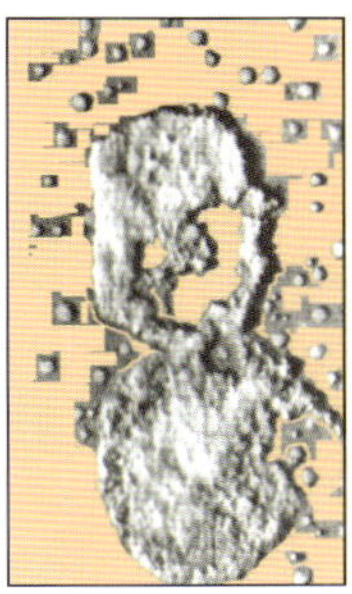

2.2b

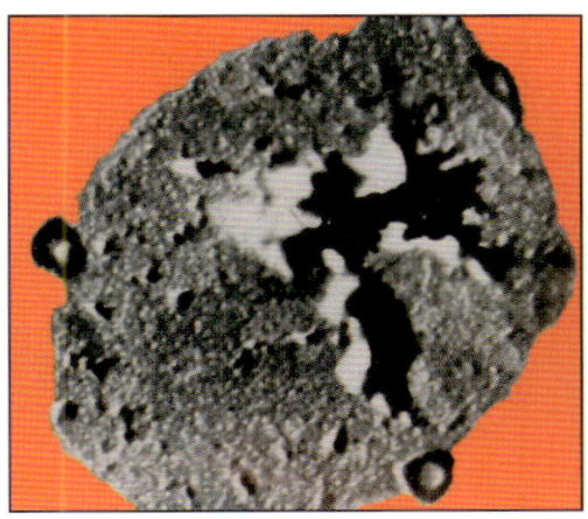

3.2b

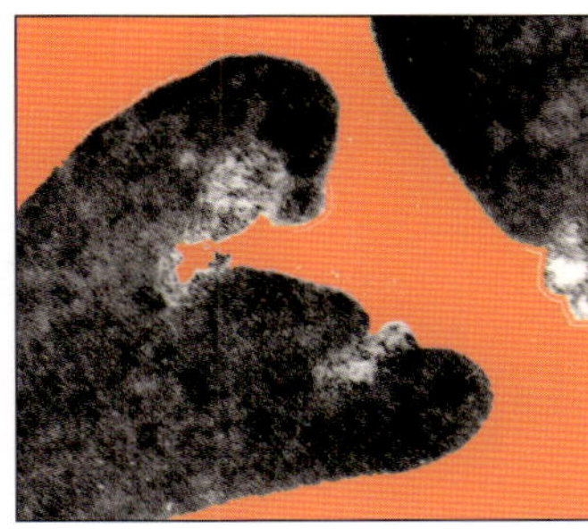

3.1b

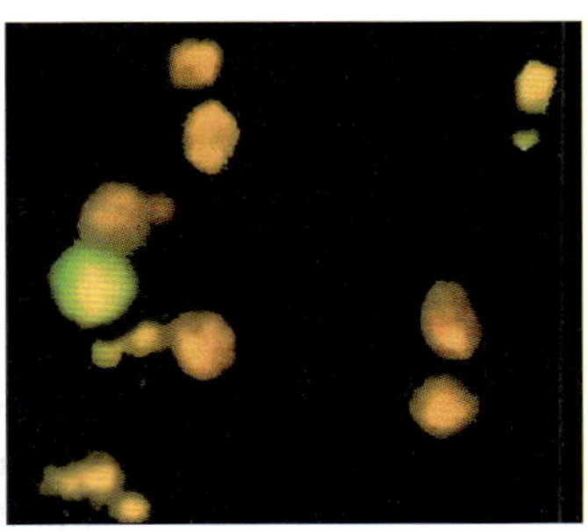

3.2a

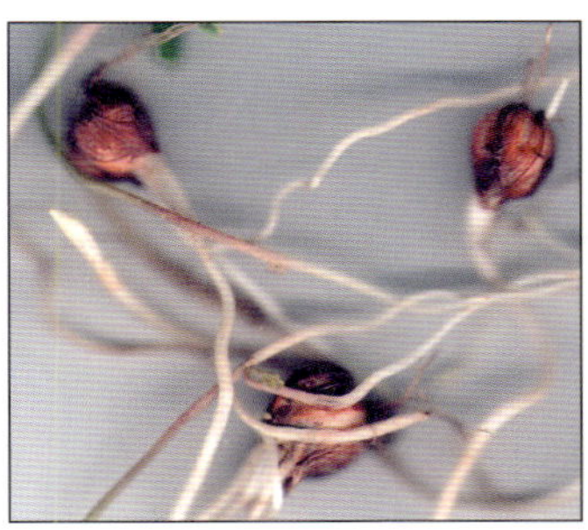

4.1*

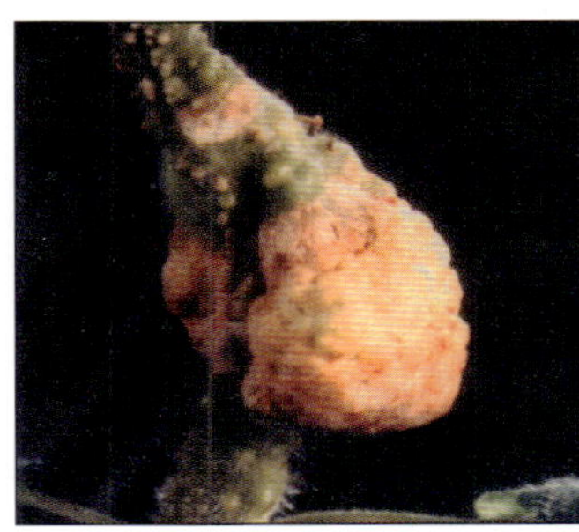

7.6*

*Figs 4.1 (Rhizobium) and 7.6 are included together for comparison purposes and to remind the reader that the difference between the benign symbiotic relationship in the case of Rhizobium and the plant, and the tumour-causing property of the same type of bacterium, is the possession by the latter of plasmid DNA.

The Step by Step Process towards Malignancy in a Section of a Plant Tumour (A After Smith) and as shown Diagrammatically in Leukaemia (B After Greaves)

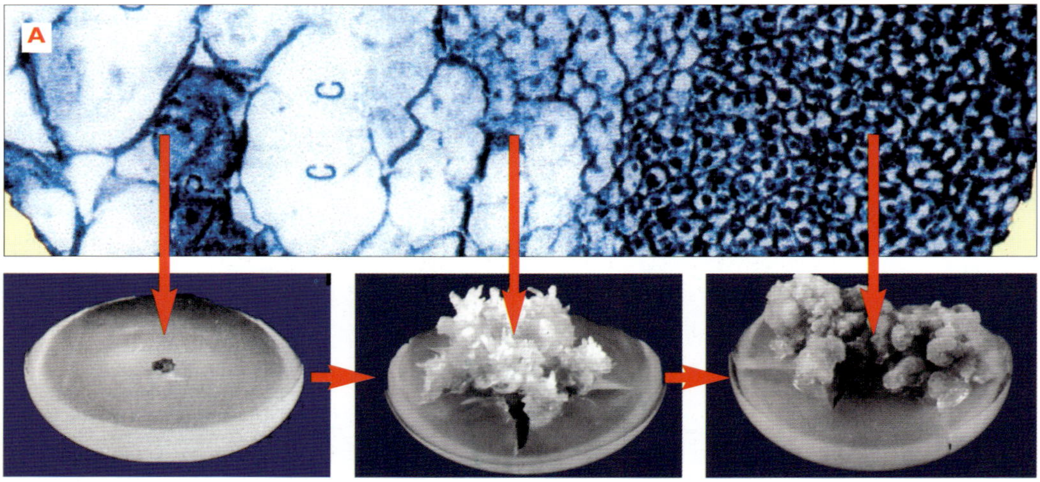

Progression to Malignancy is accompanied by the gradual ability to grow on artificial medium containing minimal growth materials both in plant and human disease (Chapter 7)

B

Fig. 7.3 Clonal Selection and Cellular Phenotypes in Leukaemia

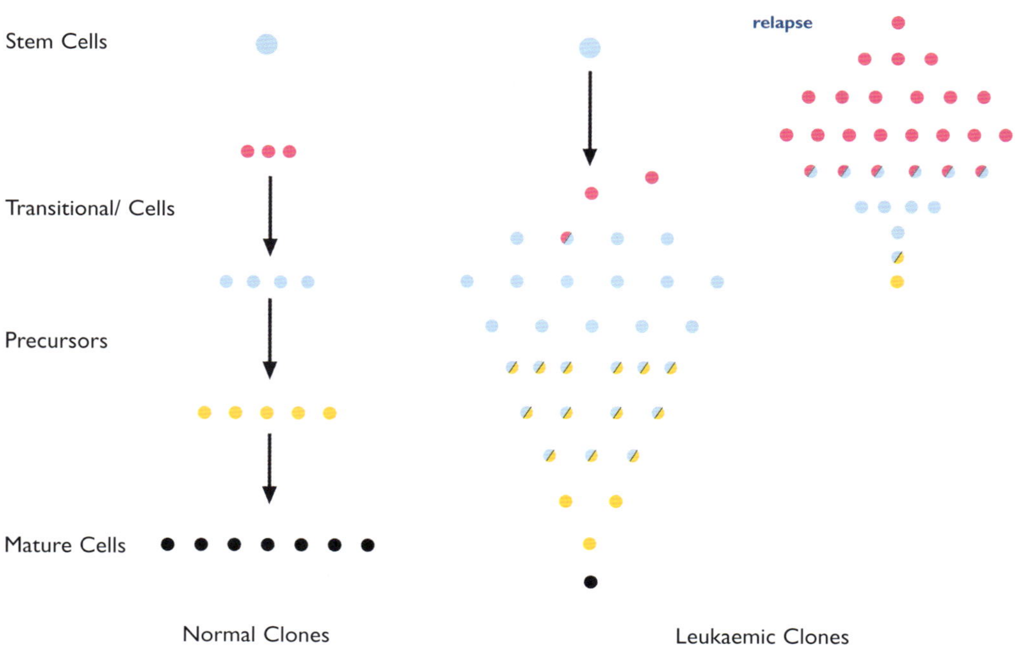

Chromosome painting (Fig. 7.7) and the acid-fast 'Mother Cells' characteristic of the Human Bacterial Parasite (7.9)

7.7a

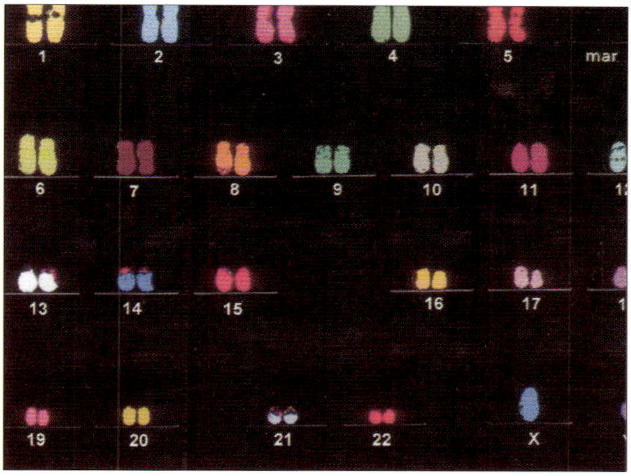

7.7b

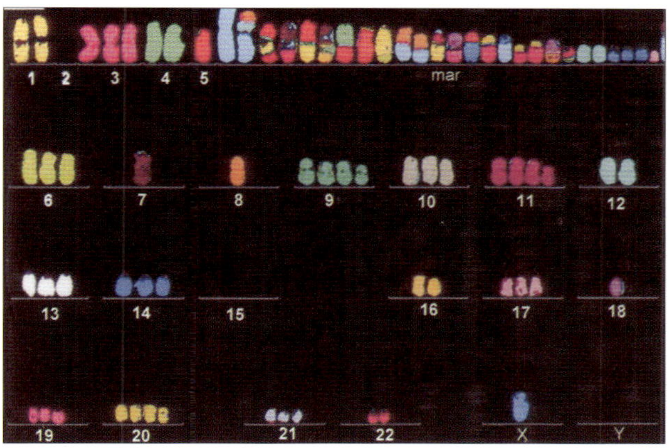

7.9 Large acid fast rods stained red

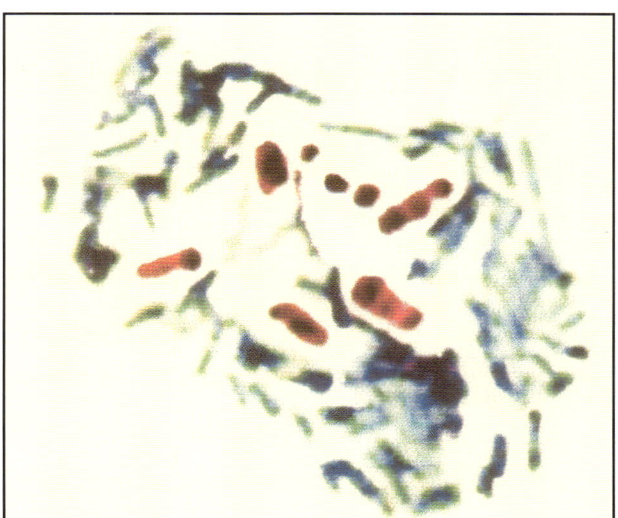

Selected Images from Chapters 8 and 9 and Appendix 2

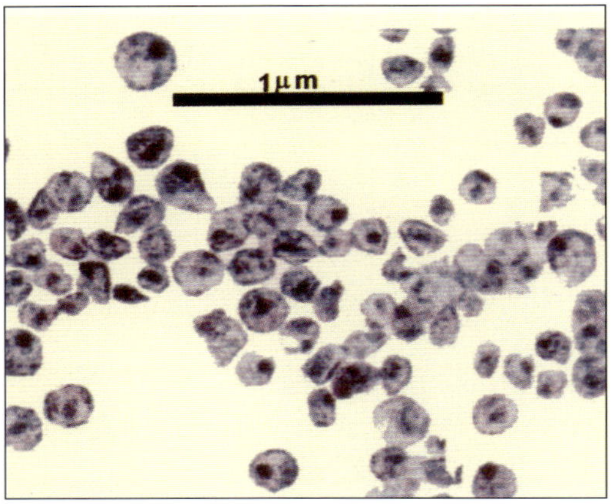

8.6a

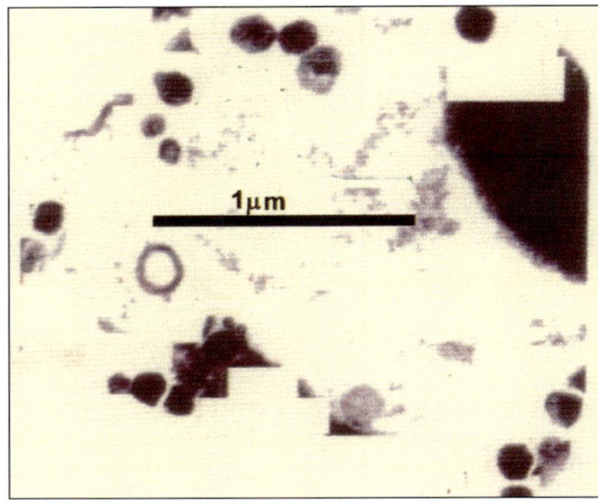

8.6b

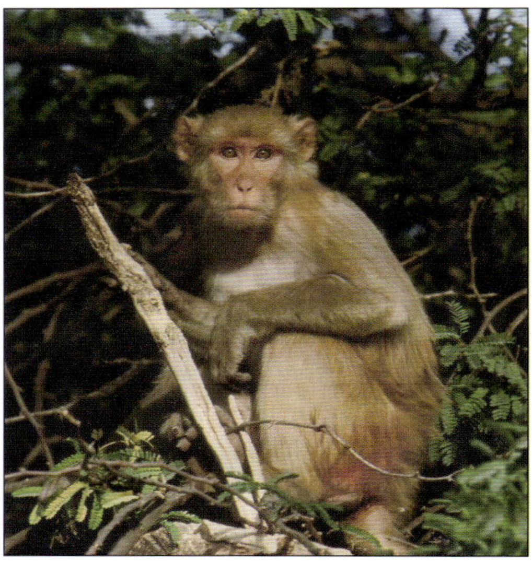

9.5

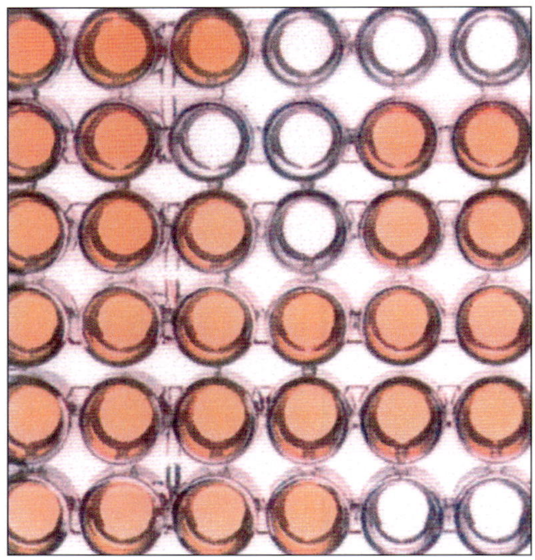

9.2 Elisa

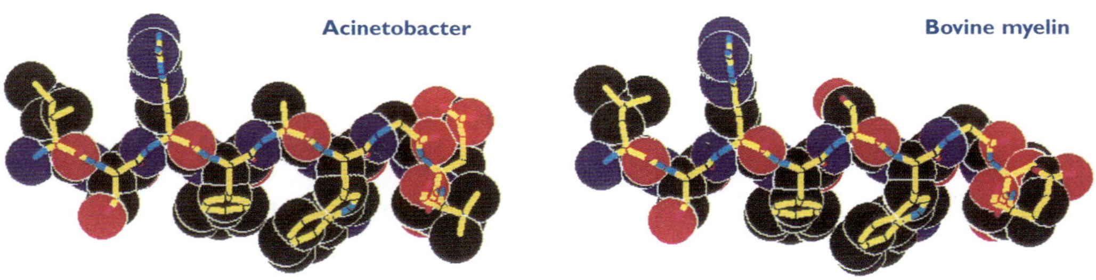

Molecular mimicry Appendix 2

tumours. However, in the case of the leukaemias, unlike the plant situation, it is not easy to determine the timing of the early stages. Chromosome abnormalities such as the Ph chromosome can provide a diagnosis for the relatively early stages of some types of leukaemia (CML in adults and ALL in infants < 1 yr and children 2-10 yrs) but how much it is a cause and how much an effect of some other factor is still not known for certain. As already mentioned, the Ph chromosome is regarded as evidence of a 'first hit' and occurrence of a 'second hit' is manifested by the appearance of further chromosome abnormalities in patients going into a blast crisis.

However, recent studies have shown that some chromosome abnormalities are initiated *in utero* and these studies have provided a considerable amount of information on several fronts. The abnormalities have consisted mainly of translocations, and the resulting 'chimeric genes' are excellent indicators for prognosis and therapy. The fact that it has been unequivocally demonstrated that they occur before birth is of immense interest especially in view of the possible relevance of maternal to foetal transfer of infective agents and of microchimerism (Chapter Nine).

The first investigations (Ford *et al* 1993) were made on monozygotic twins who were concordant for infant leukaemia. In most cases of this condition there is a translocation between chromosome 11q23, the relevant gene being called variously MLL ALL-1, HTRX or HRX, and one of several partner chromosomes. Interestingly in the present context of a biological viewpoint, the gene in question shares homology with the *Drosophila* gene trithorax, which is a developmental gene. Normally individual patients have break-points at different places but in this study three pairs of infant twins with concordant leukaemia shared the same rearrangement, thus showing not only that there had been intra-placental 'metastasis' but also that the chromosome event had happened *in utero*.

Further studies (Gale *et al* 1997) confirmed that leukaemia could be initiated prenatally in young children. This was achieved by retrospective inspection, using PCR, of neonatal blood spots (Guthrie cards) taken routinely by heel prick at birth for the presence of leukaemic cells and comparing them with those occurring in patients with acute lymphoblastic leukaemia at ages of five months to two years. The finding of unique MLL-AF4 fusion sequences in the blood spots provided indisputable evidence that the aberrant cells had arisen during pregnancy, thus opening up an important research pathway. It is now clear that there are several subsets of leukaemias and that some groups segregate with age and in prognosis.

Additional studies have emphasized the need for at least two 'hits' in the development of leukaemia. A study on six hundred blood samples from unselected neonates showed a 1% occurrence of a leukaemic TEL-AML-1 fusion gene, and since this represents 100 times the risk of acute lymphoblastic leukaemia, the finding clearly indicates that progression to malignancy of this supposed pre-leukaemic clone is a rare event, and points to the need for a second 'hit' after birth which manifests itself in the form of further chromosome and/or molecular abnormalities. It is estimated that an *in utero* hit can give rise to overt leukaemia up to at least fourteen years later (Greaves 2002).

INFECTION AND/OR IRRADIATION IN CHILDHOOD LEUKAEMIA

Whilst recent studies have been directed towards investigating environmental chemical agents as possible causes for the *in utero* first hits (Alexander *et al* 2001), searches for significant infective agents have been carried out for as long as leukaemia has been recognised as a disease entity, although it has never seriously been regarded as a conventional infectious condition.

The finding of disease clusters (mini-epidemics) has been a long-established sign of some sort of a function of an infective agent, and in our laboratory for example we investigated a cluster of Crohn's disease that occurred in a Cotswold village (Allan *et al* 1986). Disease clusters are detected by statistical analyses *i.e.* comparing the excess incidence of disease with the expected incidence and since the early 1980's there has been some concern about the fact that clusters of leukaemias were being detected near nuclear installations. The most well-known ones in the UK were close to the nuclear complex sites at Sellafield in the north of England and Dounreay in the extreme north of Scotland.

In brief, it was thought that the blood cancer clusters near Sellafield and Dounreay could be due to man-made radiation from the nuclear complex; paternal pre-conception exposure to ionising radiations, or to some kind of infective process occurring because of population mixing with the influx of a new workers employed at the power plants.

Generally speaking, investigations into the possible effect of radiation from the Sellafield plant in particular concluded that the increases in the case numbers were unlikely to be related to local pollution from nuclear waste. The idea that paternal exposure to irradiation might be responsible for the increased incidence in their children was also dismissed and it was generally accepted that some other explanation needed to be sought (Doll *et al* 1994).

The third suggestion - the one that is most relevant in the present context - that an infective agent is involved in leukaemia - was based on classical epidemiological reasoning, the well-known fact that populations in geographically isolated areas are particularly susceptible to infectious agents e.g. measles, that are controllable in other areas where the agent is widespread in the populace. In order to test this hypothesis the nuclear installation factor had to be taken out of the equation.

Accordingly Kinlen (1988) investigated an appropriate population in a 'new town' - Glenrothes in central Fife - similar to Seascale and Dounreay in being an isolated place, nowhere near nuclear installations but which had undergone large population influxes, and he did discover a significant excess of leukaemia deaths in that population.

This fulfilled the various aspects of the hypothesis; that influxes of population into rural and isolated areas are conducive to epidemics of certain infections; that Sellafield and Dounreay are extreme examples of isolation and population influx and that some unidentified virus (or viruses) can cause childhood leukaemia. Retroviruses seemed likely candidates at the time - agents that purportedly could be widely present in a population but causing illness only in a small percentage of the population (Chapter Five).

The idea that these observations could indicate the involvement of an infective agent in the aetiology of leukaemia has been followed up by several workers e.g. Greaves and Alexander (1993), in a discussion paper about the possible involvement of infective agents in childhood ALL, agreed that relative isolation, combined with population mixing, could have a role in micro-epidemics of leukaemia in children.

Some of these studies have indicated that *in utero* exposure may be significant (Petridou *et al* 1996, Dickinson and Parker 1999) supposedly causing the 'first hit' mentioned above. However, assessments of the relationship between clusters of cases of leukaemias and the relevance of nuclear installations in the vicinity are notoriously difficult to make and are well outside the scope of this book.

A recent publication (Laurier *et al* 2002) provides a balanced account of the current position on the leukaemia-clustering/nuclear plant phenomena, mentioning the more recent reports concerning those that have been reported in France at the La Hague reprocessing plant and in Germany at the Krummel power plant in addition to the most well-known ones referred to above.

The situation has been considerably complicated by the degree of media interest and suggestions of cover-ups in some cases, but the general view is that proximity to nuclear stations is only a negligible factor in the causing of the leukaemia clusters, compared with the effects of natural background irradiation and possible fallout from nuclear accidents and weapon testing.The population mixing aspect, with the concomitant belief in some sort of infective agent, albeit of uncertain provenance (Darby and Roman 1996), seems still to be regarded as the more relevant factor.

SOLID TUMOURS AS LATER STAGES IN CANCER PROGRESSION

It will be recalled that Nowell (1976) believed that solid tumours are usually a late clonal development, and the as already mentioned chromosome abnormalities - the hallmark of the cancerous cell - are abundant at this stage. In fact, chromosome abnormalities in solid tumours have been much more difficult to analyse than those in the leukaemias and until recently such studies have not been very successful.

However, the development of ingenious techniques of chromosome 'painting' and genomic hybridisation have revolutionised this area of study in recent years. Genetic genomic hybridisation (GGH) allows comparisons to be made between genomic changes in primary tumours and those in established cell-lines.This complements the technique of multicoloured chromosome painting in the investigation of cell-lines, which permits a more detailed examination than that provided by fresh tumour material. In the chromosome 'painting' technique - spectral karyotyping SKY - each of the twenty four human chromosomes can be made to appear differently coloured and this can provide fascinating and informative images of chromosome rearrangements in colorectal and breast tumour cell-lines which appear to provide good models of the corresponding primary tumours. (Schrock *et al* 1996, Davidson *et al* 2000)

Abdel-Rahman *et al* (2001) investigated chromosome rearrangements in 17 colorectal cancer derived cell-lines shown to be representative of those found in primary tumours using (SKY) in combination with CGH. The results, which are too esoteric to be discussed here in detail, demonstrated at least three karyotypes which between them revealed a large array of abnormalities, including multiple unbalanced and balanced translocations, replication errors (RER) and in some cases a tendency to triploidy (3 chromosomes in the place of 2).

Fig 7.7 'Chromosome Painting' in Cancer Research

a)

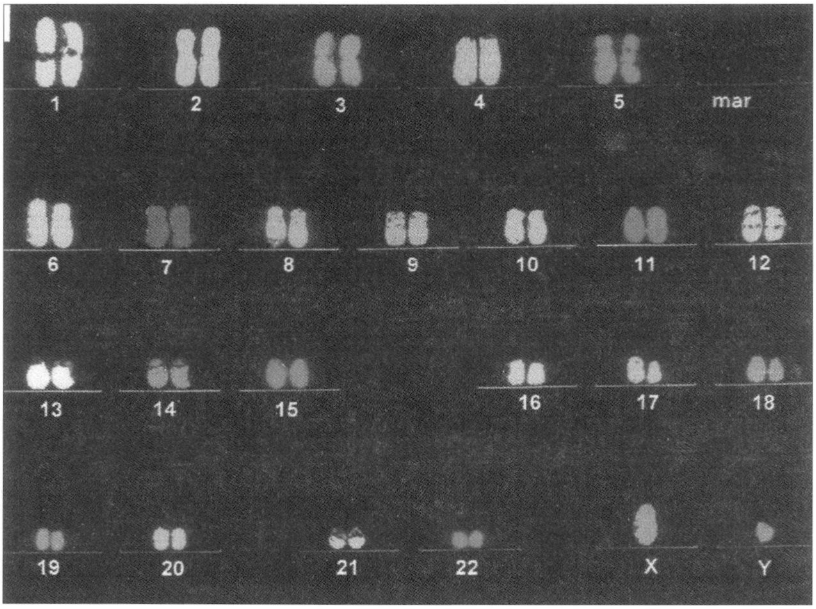

b)

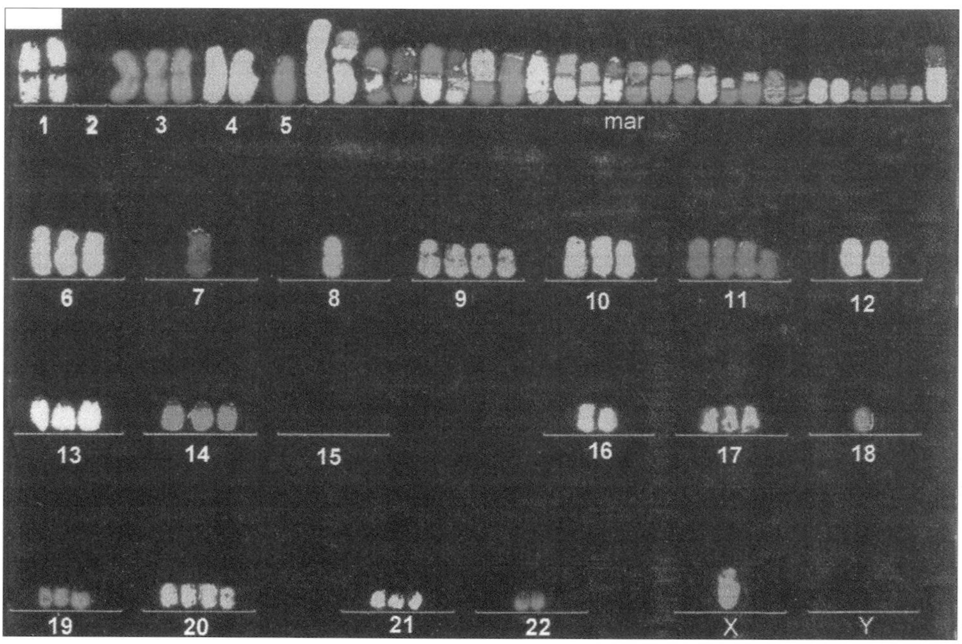

Fig. 7.7a The chromosome composition of a normal cell using a 'chromosome painting' technique, which is in marked contrast to that of
Fig. 7.7b This was prepared from a breast cancer cell (after the acquirement of resistance to puromycin) and is highly abnormal, with extra chromosomes, lost copies of others and many composed of fused pieces of different chromosomes. Reproduced by kind permission of Peter Duesberg and Li Ruhong.

Similar analyses of breast cancer cell-lines were carried out by Davidson *et al* (2000) who examined nineteen breast carcinoma cell-lines and one normal breast epithelial cell-line in their capacity as model examples of chromosome rearrangements in breast carcinomas. CGH profiles were compared with those of 106 primary breast cancers and good correlations were found. The cell-lines varied from being perfectly diploid to being highly aneuploid, the latter tending to fall into two groups; one that steadily lost chromosomes and the other that steadily gained them, together with other abnormalities. Translocations were varied and 98% were unbalanced. The most frequently involved chromosome was 8, and further work along these lines has concentrated on translocations on those with breakpoints at 8p12 (Courtney-Cahen *et al* 2000).

RSV/src AS A MODEL FOR HUMAN CANCER

As explained in Chapter Five the *onc*-retroviruses are ones in which the gene responsible for the cancer-causing property of the viruses is actually derived from a former host cell *e.g.* in the case of the Rous Sarcoma Virus (RSV), the *onc* gene originated in the nuclear material of a chicken. This model has been used with respect to human cancer by two authorities on the subject, each of whom presents an essentially pessimistic view in this regard inasmuch as each regards the human cancer process to be the result of sometimes unavoidable environmental factors and ultimately of bad luck. This pessimism is in complete contrast to the hopes that the model could provide leads that in due course would provide a vaccine against human cancer discussed earlier.

Duesberg believes that *onc*-retroviruses provide a model for human cancer by virtue of the fact that their cancer-producing potential relies on the 'illegitimate' fusion of host cellular genes and suggests that human cancer results from a similar process. However, he judges that the straight *onc*-retrovirus model represents a phenomenon which statistically verges on the edge of extreme improbability and considers the recombination of cell-control genes *in situ* to be a much more probable scenario for cancer-formation. The aneuploidy that such fusions would produce, he maintains, would be sufficient to cause cancer - one of the pathways being the inactivation of certain growth control genes (such as p53 in the light of today's knowledge). (Ruhong *et al* 1997)

Greaves (2001) sees the retrovirus model as paralleling the step by step process of mutations in growth control genes that in the process of Darwinian selection lead eventually to cancer in humans. He provided a good analogy for this situation when he compared the virus containing the normal cellular genes hijacked from the original host (e.g. chicken or mouse), with a Trojan horse, the contents of the horse being the same class of genes as those cellular ones that are mutated in human cancer cells.

In the case of the Trojan horse/virus model, alien growth control genes bring about the growth control anarchy in one step.

BACTERIA AS ALTERNATIVE VECTORS OF ALIEN GROWTH-CONTROLLING DNA

The mechanism of tumour formation in plants, as a model for human cancer, has received very little attention, but interest has been re-stimulated by the discovery of similarities in neo-vascularization. The basic mechanism and general characteristics of plant and human cancers have strong similarities as already discussed.

The interpretation of this model is that some human cancers result from the integration of DNA from one human into another, the Trojan horse in this case being a bacterium (Pease 1990). The most obvious candidate for this is the human endoparasite already referred to.

THE HUMAN BACTERIAL ENDOPARASITE

There are many reports in the literature of a gram positive bacterium from the blood and body fluids of human subjects in disorders normally regarded as non-infective, or from normal subjects; and many claims have been made that there is a causative relationship between the bacteria and clonal disorders including cancer and arthritis. Accurate descriptions of the life-cycle of this organism have been published on several occasions for over a century, some showing several phases of a life-cycle and some showing fewer phases but easily recognisable descriptions. These were listed by the contributors to the meeting held in New York in November 1969 to which I have already referred.

One of the problems, apart from the diversion caused by the discovery of RT, which led to the fruitless search for a retroviral cause of human cancer (Chapter Five) in gaining acceptance for this work, was the difficulty presented in classifying the bacterium.

This was largely due to the fact that computerised numerical methods for the purposes had been adopted only a few years before and still had all the appeal of being 'state of the art' technology. As I mentioned in Chapter Four, these techniques are excellent when it comes to analysing strains of bacteria already recognised as being related, which need further studies to determine differences at the level of strains of bacteria, but are of little use at a higher level.

The computer-programs do not take account in any significant way of the life-cycles of organisms. In the situation under discussion, the ability to pass through a life-cycle is essential since the bacteria need to exist, not only in close symbiotic, parasitic or pathogenic relation with their human or plant hosts, but also outside the host where they need to be able to withstand 'the vicissitudes of life', as discussed in Chapter One.

Bisset (1962) put the computer philosophy succinctly when he wrote:

'the machines are the new fundamentalists and if we ask for their assistance, we must play their game according to their rules. Adamson had protested that nobody is entitled to claim some characters as important and others as secondary. All characters are of equal importance and all must be accorded equal weight......... Fundamentalists are, of course, entitled to their opinions but now that calculating machines are coming, so to speak, to their assistance, our cosy biological family life is in danger of being broken up. I think this is one occasion when we should stand firm and tell the machines to mind their own business and go back to deciding for ourselves what we want to think is important'.

This unsophisticated reliance on the part of many investigators on numerical analysis techniques was exacerbated by the *idée fixe* that medical and agricultural bacteriology were two entirely different areas. In fact as I have already pointed out the basic patterns of human and animal cancers are similar, a fact highlighted by the recent discovery by Roni Aloni and his colleagues of neo-vascularization - the equivalent of angiogenesis - in the formation of plant tumours.

In our laboratory, even though it was situated in a medical school, this traditional division was disregarded and work on life-cycles of *Rhizobium*, which were regarded as a specialised sporing bacillus (Bisset 1952, Gillberg 1969), was carried out intermittently over several years. The resemblance of the cancer isolates, particularly the 'mother cell' phases was striking.

The discovery of the *modus operandi* of plant cancer in the mid 1970s seemed to provide the final piece of the jigsaw and supported the view expressed much earlier by Erwin Smith - the discoverer of *A tumefaciens* - that the cause of human cancer would prove to be similar to that of plant cancer.

Fig 7.8a The Human Bacterial Parasite

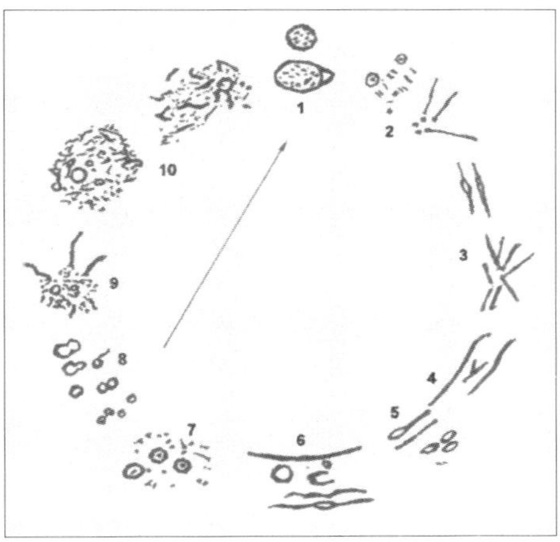

Fig. 7.8a Diagram of the life-cycle of an organism consistently isolated from blood and tumours of cancer patients and animals (Alexander-Jackson, 1954).

(1) Cysts or 'spore-sacs' filled with acid-fast bodies, 2-4µm in size. (2) Acid-fast bodies sprouting hair-like filaments. (3) Needle-like rods with pointed ends. (4) Larger rods, which may become motile. (5) Spore-like bodies. (6) Filaments and ring forms. (7) Minute acid-fast bodies (0.2µm). (8) Globoidal bodies, 0.5-2.0µm, sometimes refractile. (9) and (10) Zoogleal matrix forms or symplasms.

Fig 7.8b The Parasite Demonstrated by Various Techniques from a Variety of Sources

a)

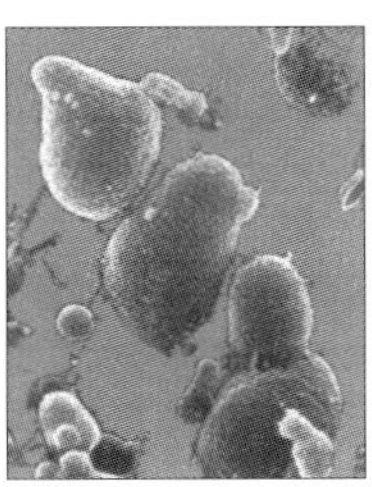

b)

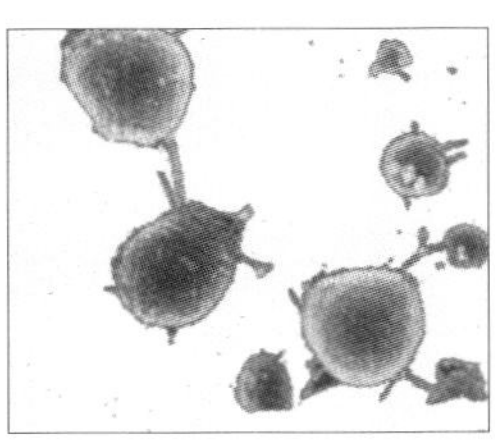

c)

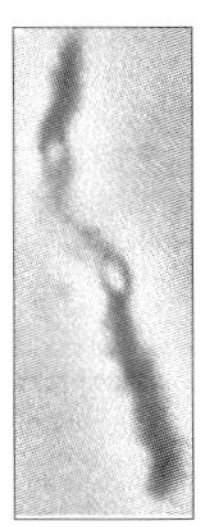

a) and b) show cyst-like forms corresponding to stage 1 in the cycle depicted by Alexander-Jackson. a) was isolated from a laboratory culture of *A. tumefaciens*, b) was isolated from a leukaemia patient (SEM).
c) shows spore-like bodies within a filament isolated from a patient with Crohn's Disease equivalent to stages 4-6 in the cycle (Phase contrast).

d)

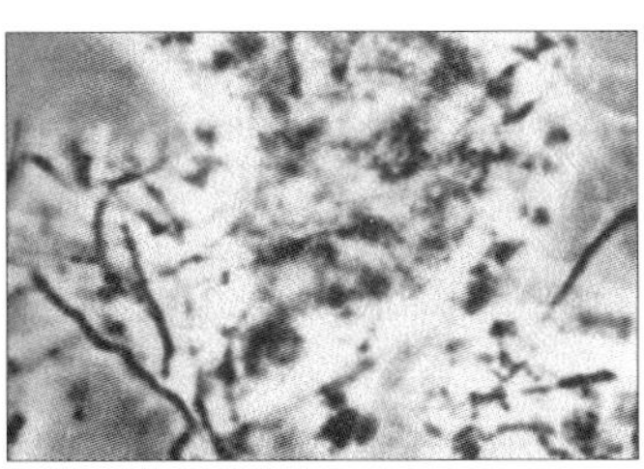

e)

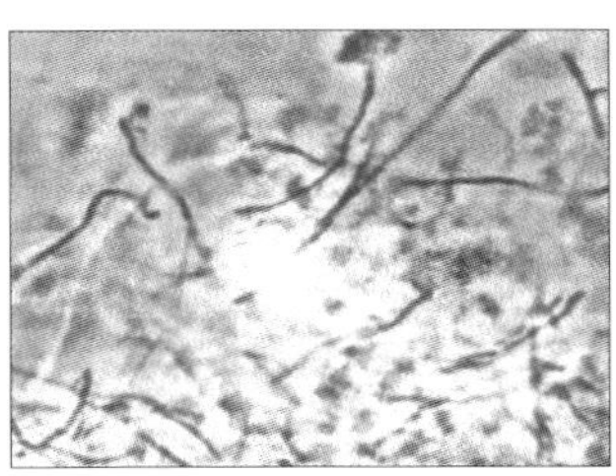

d) and e) are equivalent to stages 9 and 10 and show filaments arising from the symplasm. The isolates were derived from a patient with Crohn's Disease.

We have accumulated results such as these over a period of some 20 years and it must be remembered that the parasite exists in healthy and diseased subjects. I have thus chosen to illustrate the bacteria in their various stages from a variety of sources. (Pease 1989, Pease and Tallack 1990).

One of the most outstanding features of the endoparasite is the occurrence of large acid-fast bodies illustrated in Fig. 7.9. Alexander-Jackson discovered these in isolates from cancer patients after her first depiction of the life-cycle. We found these forms independently, initially in RA patients, and to us the resemblance to *Rhizobium* (*A. tumefaciens* minus the Ti plasmid - Chapter Four) was clear.

Fig 7.9 Acid-fast Mother Cells of the Bacterial Parasite

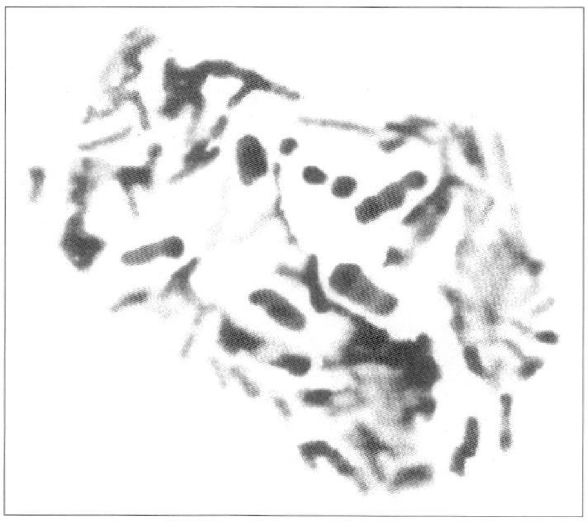

Fig. 7.9 A preparation stained by a modified Ziehl-Neelsen (ZN) stain showing characteristic acid-fast mother cells of the human endoparasite, which resemble those found in *Rhizobium* (Chapter Four). This particular preparation was made from the synovial fluid from a patient with Rheumatoid Arthritis (RA - Chapter Nine). Alexander-Jackson demonstrated these same elements in cancer patients at the N.Y. Symposium in 1969 (Chapters Eight and Nine).

It is outside the scope of this book to go into detail about what is essentially a problem of bacterial taxonomy. Useful references concerning this can be found in the N.Y. Acad. Sci. 174 1969; Bisset and Hale 1951; Bisset 1952; Bisset 1959 and Gillberg 1969.

Fig 7.10 The Proposed *Modus Operandi* (MO) of Some Human Cancers

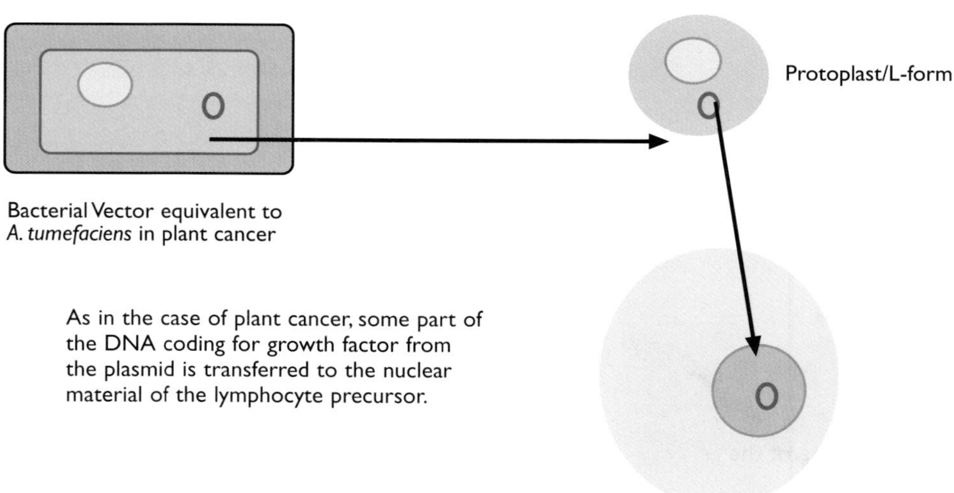

The proposed mechanism shown in Fig. 7.10 is basically similar to that proposed by Greaves for a putative viral cause of leukaemia starting in the bone marrow, but in this case the proposed agent is a cell wall deficient bacterial form containing DNA coding for growth factors. If the host cell is successfully colonised, the potential for malignancy is then in place. This would essentially be equivalent to the 'mutator' cell envisaged by Loeb, and effectively the whole package for malignancy is in this 'mutator' cell. Other cells may well be infected initially, but the likelihood is that in accordance with the current view of the progression to malignancy in humans, eventually particular descendent clones will become predominant.

Where infection occurs in solid tissue it is envisaged that again, one originally infected cell will give rise to a particularly successful clone and in due course give rise to the high degree of chromosome aberrations that usually characterise advanced solid tumours.

In fact, after the initiation of the 'mutator' cell the stages and their mechanisms would not differ from the standard model; however, the infection itself is external. The mechanism of this seems likely to be parenteral, the most likely route being the maternal to child one, although blood transfusion cannot be ruled out. Clearly, however, numerous hurdles exist blocking the way to the onset of malignancy.

The immense variability in individual cancers can in this model be accounted for to some extent by the characteristics of the alien DNA - the amount and virulence and extent of colonisation - as well as by the individual features of the defence mechanisms, exposure to carcinogens and other environmental features and of course to inherited predisposing mutations.

The evidence of the possibility of the involvement of infective agents in leukaemia inferred from observations of clusters near nuclear power facilities as a result of the attendant population mixing does not appear to have a significant bearing on the proposed model.

As far as the effect of irradiation is concerned, it seems probable that it is only in the case of accidents such as that at Chernobyl that any effect on the occurrence of leukaemia can be relevant. Conceivably in cases of accidents, irradiation could act as a 'second hit'.

In the next chapter the suggestion made that RSV is a CWD bacterial form is reappraised, and this is of interest in the cancer situation because it would suggest that the CWD form of the bacterial parasite is the human equivalent of the RSV causative agent of chicken cancer.

SUMMARY

In this chapter it is argued that notwithstanding the differences between animals and plants the basic nature of cancer is essentially the same in both groups. At the start of the process a cell gains an advantage over its fellows by evading the normal growth controls so that it can proliferate freely. Then by a step by step process, changes in cellular structure and differentiation, accompanied by a progressive loss of the reliance on normal growth factors and hormones, occur.

Furthermore it is indicated that the vascular system so important in the human disease is also of importance in cancer progression in plants. It is also argued that taking into account the various characteristics of human cancers, including heritable factors, chromosome aberrations and the effects of irradiation, and bearing in mind the *onc/src* retrovirus model of chicken cancer model that a case can be made for the bacteria associated with human cancers and resembling *Agrobacterium tumefaciens* acting in a way analogous to those causing plant cancer, by allowing alien DNA to enter human cell nuclei thereby interfering with the growth cell mechanisms.

REFERENCES

Abdel-Rahman, W.M. Katsura, K. Rens, W. *et al* (2001) Spectral karyotyping suggests additional subsets of colorectal cancers characterised by pattern of chromosome rearrangement
Proc. Natl. Acad. Sci. USA 98 2538-2543

Alexander, F.E., Patheal, S.L., Biondi, A. (2001) Transplacental Chemical Exposure and Risk of Infant Leukaemia with MLL Gene Fusion
Cancer Research 61 2542-2546

Allan, R.N., Pease, P and Ibbotson (1986) Clustering of Crohn's Disease in a Cotswold Village
Quarterly Journal of Medicine 299 473-478

Aloni, R., Wolf, A. Avni, A. *et al* (1998) The Never Ripe Mutant Provides Evidence that Tumour-Induced Ethylene Controls the Morphogenesis of Agrobacterium tumefaciens-Induced Crown Galls on Tomato Stems
Plant Physiol 117 841-849

Baker, S.J. Markowitz, S Fearon, E.R. *et al* (1990) Suppression of Human Colorectal Carcinoma Cell Growth by Wild-Type p53
Science 245 912-915

Bisset, K.A., and Hale, C.M.F (1951) The Production of Swarmers in *Rhizobium* spp.
J Gen. Microbiol. 5 592-595

Bisset, K.A. (1952) Complete and reduced life-cycles in *Rhizobium.*
J Gen. Microbol. 7 233-242

Bisset, K.A. (1959) Some Characteristics of *Rhizobium* Strains from Tropical Legumes.
J Gen. Microbiol. 20 89-90

Bisset, K.A. (1962) The New Fundamentalists
The Listener

Boveri, T. (1914) *Zur Frage der Enstehung Maligner Tumoren*
Gustav Fischer Verlag Jena Germany

Braun, A.C. (1965) The Reversal of Tumour Growth.
Sci. Am. 213 No. 5

Courtney-Cahen, C., Morris, J.S. and Edwards, P.A.W. (2000) Chromosome Translocations in Breast Cancer with Breakpoints at 8p12
Genomics 66 15-25

Darby, S.C. and Roman, E. (1996) Links in childhood leukaemia
Nature 382 303-304

Davidson, J.M., Gorringe, K.L., Chin, S-F. *et al* (2000) Molecular cytogenetic analysis of breast cancer cell lines
British Journal of Cancer 83 1309-1317

Dickinson, H.O. and Parker L. (1999) Quantifying the effect of population mixing on childhood leukaemia risk: the Seascale cluster
Br. J Cancer 81 144-151

Doll, R., Evans, H.J. and Darby, S. (1994) Parental exposure not to blame
Nature 367 678-680

Duesberg, P.H. (1983) Retroviral transforming genes in normal cells?
Nature 304 219-26

Ford, A.M., Ridge, S. Cabrera, M.E. (1993) *In utero* rearrangements in the trithorax-related oncogene in infant leukaemias
Nature 362 358-360

Gale, K.B., Ford, A.M. Repp, R. (1997) Backtracking leukaemia to birth: Identification of clonotypic gene fusion sequences in neonatal blood spots
Proc. Natl. Acad Sci USA 94 13950-13954

Gillberg, B (1969) Heat Resistance and Pigmented Variants of *Rhizobium*.
Nature 222 574-575

Greaves, M and Alexander, F.E. (1993) An infectious Aetiology for Common Acute Lymphoblastic Leukaemia in Childhood
Leukaemia 7 349-360

Greaves, M. (1997) Stem cells, haemopoiesis and leukaemia. in Introduction to the Cellular and Molecular Biology of Cancer 3rd Ed. Editors L.M. Franks and N.M. Teich
Oxford University Press

Greaves, M. (2001) Cancer, the evolutionary legacy
Oxford University Press
Greaves, M. (2002) Childhood leukaemia
B.M.J. 324 283-287

Hupp, T.R., Lane, D.P. and Ball, K.L. (2000) Strategies for manipulating the p53 pathway in the treatment of human cancer
Biochem. J. 352 1-17

Kinlen, L. (1988) Evidence for an Infective cause of childhood leukaemia:: Comparison of a Scottish New Town with Nuclear Reprocessing Sites in Britain
Lancet Dec 10 1323-1327

Kinlen, L.J. (1995) Epidemiological evidence for an infective basis in childhood leukaemia
Br. J Cancer 71 1-5

Kinzler, K.W. and Volgelstein, B. (1998) Landscaping the Cancer Terrain
Science 280 1036

Laurier, D. Grosche, B and Hall, P. (2002) Risk of Childhood Leukaemia in the vicinity of Nuclear Installations
Acta Oncologia 41 14-24

Levine, A.J. (1997) p53, the cellular gatekeeper for growth and division
Cell 88 323-331

Livingstone, V. and Alexander-Jackson, E. (1970) A specific type of micro-organism cultivated from malignancy: bacteriology and proposed classification.
Ann. N.Y. Acad Sci. 174 636-654

Loeb, L.A. (2001) A mutator phenotype in cancer
Cancer Res. 61 3230-3239

Marx, J. (2002) Debate Surges Over the Origins of Genomic Defects in Cancer
Science 297 544-5

Malkin, D. Frederick, P. Strong, L. *et al* (1990) Germ Line p53 Mutations in a Familial Syndrome of Breast Cancer, Sarcomas and Other Neoplasms
Science 250 1233-1238

Nowell, P.C. (1976) The Clonal Evolution of Tumour Cell Population
Science 194 23-28

Pease, P.(1970) Discussion: Microorganisms Associated with Malignancy
Ann. N.Y. Acad Sci 174 782-784

Pease, P.E. (1990) The widespread bacterial endoparasitism in man and its possible role in malignant and autoimmune disease
Endocytobiology IV 4th International Colloquium on Endocytobiology and Symbiosis INRA Paris
Eds Nardon, P., Gianinazzi-Pearson, V., Grenier, A.M., Margulis, L. and D.C.Smith
Petridou, E. Revinthi, K. Alexander, F.E. *et al* (1996) Space-time clustering of childhood leukaemia in Greece: evidence supporting a viral aetiology.
Br.J Cancer 73 1278-1283

Pease, Phyllis E. and Tallack, Janice E. (1990) A permanent endoparasite of man I The silent zoogleal/symplasm/L-form phase
Microbios 64 173-180

Petridou, E., Trichpoulos, D. Dessypris, N. *et al* (1996) Infant leukaemia after in utero exposure to radiation from Chernobyl
Nature 382 352-353

Ruhong, L., Yerganian, G. Duesberg, P. *et al* (1997) Aneuploidy correlated 100% with chemical transformation of Chinese hamster cells
Proc Natl Acad Sci USA 94 14506-14511

Schrock, E.. du Manoir, T. Veldman, T. *et al* (1996) Multicolour Spectral Karyotyping of Human Chromosomes typing
Science 273 494-497

Schwalm, K., Aloni, R. and Langhans, M. *et al* (2003) Flavonoid-related regulation of auxin accumulation in *Agrobacterium tumefaciens*-induced plant tumours
Planta 218 163-178

Smith, E.F. (1907) On Some Resemblances of Crown-Gall to Human Cancer
Science 25 671-673

Smith, E.F. (1916) Further evidence that Crown Gall of Plants is Cancer
Science 43 871-889

Smith, E. F, (1922) Appositional Growth in Crown-Gall Tumours and in Cancers
Journal of Cancer Research 7 1-49

Tomlinson, I. and Bodmer, W. (1999) Selection, the mutation rate and cancer: Ensuring that the tail does not wag the dog
Nature America Inc. 5 11-12

Tomlinson, I., Sasieni, P. and Bodmer, W. (2002) How Many Mutations in a Cancer?
American Journal of Pathology 160 755-758

Ullrich, I.C. and Aloni, R. (2000) Vascularization is a general requirement for growth of plant and animal tumours
Journal of Experimental Botany 51 1951-1960

Veselov, D., Langhans, M. and Hartung, W. *et al* (2003) Development of *Agrobacterium tumefaciens* C-58-induced plant tumours and impact on host shoots are controlled by a cascade of jasmonic acid, auxin, cytokinin, ethylene and abscisic acid.
Planta 216 512-522

Virchow. R. (1871) *Cellular Pathology 4th ed.* Berlin, as quoted by Smith E F, (1922)

CHAPTER EIGHT

AIDS

'It is the consensus that is the problem: Scholar B accepts the routine followed by Scholar A, and Scholars C, D and E join the bandwagon, and in support they cite each other. Agreement and repetition have conferred a spurious authority on an operation which did not work (was flawed) in the first place. Remember that we set the agenda; those who follow rely on us; what we get wrong becomes the permanent heritage of the discipline.

Before building an argument be sure you understand the meaning of the materials you are working with.'

Buttrey (1994)

'We know that to err is human, but the HIV/AIDS hypothesis is one hell of a mistake.'

Mullis (1995)

INTRODUCTION 112

HISTORY OF HIV/AIDS 113

AIDS - THE BEGINNING
THE FIRST RETROVIRUS CULTURE AND THE DISCOVERY OF P24 IN AIDS
EARLY MISGIVINGS ABOUT THE ROLE OF HIV
TEN YEARS OF DISAPPOINTMENT
A WATERSHED IN AIDS RESEARCH - TEN YEARS ON
THE NEW MODEL OF VIRUS PATHOGENICITY
THE 'NEW VIEW' OF AIDS AND THE ONSET OF ANTI-RETROVIRAL THERAPY
BLOOD PRODUCT STUDIES
AIDS, HIV AND HAEMOPHILIACS
SIV VACCINE RESEARCH IN NON-HUMAN PRIMATES

HIV AND MICROBIAL CONTAMINATION 124

RETROVIRUSES AND CELLULAR CONTAMINATION 127

RETROVIRUSES IN RETROSPECT 129

BACK TO THE FUTURE
THE CASE FOR RETROVIRUSES BEING SUB-CELLULAR ELEMENTS OF BACTERIA (SBES)

SUMMARY AND CONCLUSIONS 132

INTRODUCTION

From the onset of the epidemic, the AIDS problem has been influenced by political and financial matters to a degree unprecedented in the field of medical research, and these aspects have had a considerable influence on the course the research has taken. Even some leading establishment investigators have admitted that there has been a great deal of bad research on AIDS (Wain-Hobson 1995), and there is no doubt that the early work on which the simple 'virus equals disease' concept was founded, was seriously lacking in elementary microbiological controls.

As the extent of this has become more apparent with the passing years it has added to the disquiet felt by some investigators, especially Peter Duesberg, who almost from the start of the epidemic felt that the simple 'new virus causes new disease' concept was the result of a hunch based on expediency rather than on sound judgement.

In fact, most mainstream investigators now recognise that AIDS is not a simple virus disease comparable with the great bacterial and viral epidemics of the past, but even so, research continues almost exclusively as if this were the case. There are two reasons for this - one is that most of the funding in the search for therapies and vaccines for AIDS is not only conceptually but also commercially based, which means effectively that AIDS research and HIV research are synonymous. There is thus a considerable amount of pressure on research workers to direct and interpret their findings in a way that encourages the renewal of their grants. As far as what must now be described as the third generation of investigators is concerned, this presents no difficulty because the commercialisation of science is now a fact of life, and in any case, this generation has been taught that the cause of AIDS has already been settled as a self evident truth - that things have moved on - new technology has confirmed the original work - and that anyone who does not accept it is mad, bad or both.

The second - scientifically more telling - factor is that since AIDS appears to be an infectious disease there does not seem at present to be a more persuasive explanation other than that an infective agent is involved, and currently, HIV is the only candidate.

The result of this intense concentration on HIV is that some areas of AIDS research have become very esoteric, and for many investigators, including myself, some of the research work, especially in the realms of molecular biology, has become almost impossible to follow, let alone evaluate, and seems to be very far removed from the curing and prevention of the disease. The volume of resulting publications is now so vast that it is excessively difficult to grasp anything resembling the whole of the increasingly narrowly specialised picture.

On the other hand, it is all too easy to see that the promise of effective therapy that came in the mid-nineties has not been fulfilled, and the guarantee of an effective vaccine, notoriously made in 1984 by the then US Government Health Chief, Margaret Heckler, has now disappeared into the unforeseeable future.

This is not to say that no progress has been made with the disorder itself as opposed to managing the putative viral cause. The discovery of the p24 protein - widely regarded as the definitive AIDS antigen - by Montagnier and his colleagues in Paris in 1983, which led to the development of the

'AIDS tests', represented a great step forward. The use of these tests for screening blood and blood products has lessened the transmission of AIDS *via* these products considerably, and this constitutes a real success in a generally frustrating story.

No serious investigator denies the value of the 'AIDS test/s' and it is irresponsible and mischievous to claim, as some workers have, that anyone who has serious misgivings about the true cause of AIDS would advocate the dropping of such tests. The issue is not to do with the effectiveness of such tests in the diagnosis of AIDS; it is about their exact significance.

It is the purpose of this chapter to provide a background to the AIDS problem, a considerable amount of which can now be regarded as history, and to give an account of the current situation.

In addition, it is my intention to explain how AIDS investigators have lacked a proper understanding of the materials they have been handling; that they have not realised the extent of the contamination either by microorganisms - especially those with filterable stages - or with mammalian, often human tissues (derived from the cells used to support HIV growth); that as a result HIV has been attributed with properties that belong to the materials from these other sources and that the whole edifice of AIDS research thus becomes severely undermined.

HISTORY OF HIV/AIDS

AIDS, THE BEGINNING

The outbreak of acquired immune-deficiency syndrome (AIDS) was first recognised in the early eighties in the then highly promiscuous male gay population centred in New York, San Francisco and Los Angeles. This included engaging in high-risk conduct, often in bathhouses, such as fisting and rimming, activities which encourage the further spread of the gut/venereal diseases already common in the gay population (Shilts 1987), as well as AIDS. Subsequently, the syndrome reached other populations; recreational drug users of both sexes and sadly, but predictably, recipients of blood products, remembering that in the US, blood for transfusion or for the manufacture of Factor VIII concentrate was provided from an uncontrolled 'donor' population. Likewise, the disease spread, in due course, to the babies of infected mothers.

The first indications were the occurrence of unusual, life-threatening infections, normally easily controllable by the immune system (Fig. 8.1).

Fig. 8.1 AIDS Indicator Diseases

Candidiasis - oesophageal, pulmonary

Cryptococcosis - extra-pulmonary

Cytomegalovirus - disseminated

Cryptosporidiosis - diarrhoea persisting > 1 month

Herpes simplex virus (HSV) infection
- mucocutaneous ulceration lasting > 1 month
- pulmonary, oesophageal involvement

Kaposi's sarcoma - patient < 60 years old

Primary cerebral lymphoma - patient < 13 years old

Mycobacterium avium - disseminated
Mycobacterium kansasi - disseminated

Pseudomonas carinii - pneumonia

Cerebral toxoplasmosis

After Williams *et al* 1989 (Chapter Five)

A deficiency of CD4 helper cells (Chapter Six) was found to be associated with the disorder and appeared to be the immediate cause of the symptoms. In the circumstances it seemed reasonable to conclude that a filterable (the blood products were filtered to preclude classical bacterial infection) agent, probably a virus, could be responsible, and the so-called human immunodeficiency virus (HIV) was soon incriminated as the simple and straightforward causative agent.

The evidence upon which this assumption was made was based on the philosophy that AIDS is a classical infection rather than an immunological disorder and ever since these early days, as each fact which *prima facie* would cast doubt on the idea has emerged, new amendments have had to be added to accommodate the HIV=AIDS concept. This need for constant adjustment has reinforced the views of several investigators who had had doubts about the simple answer in the first place.

THE FIRST RETROVIRUS CULTURE AND DISCOVERY OF P24 IN AIDS

The first presumed HIV strain, associated with the AIDS protein p24/25, now considered to be p24, was discovered by Montagnier and his colleagues (Barre-Sinousi *et al*) at the Pasteur Institute in Paris in 1983. The group had already had a longstanding interest in cancer viruses before the AIDS epidemic, and with increasing fears of possible contamination of blood supplies, they began to examine imported plasma for Reverse Transcriptase, in the belief then extant that this would detect a retrovirus (Montagnier 2000).

Thereafter they became interested in isolating the putative retrovirus and discovered one in an 'at risk' patient. This index patient was a thirty three year old homosexual who presented with lymphadenopathies and who was widely travelled and had had more than fifty partners per year for an unspecified time. This clearly placed him in the classic 'at risk' category.

The virus was identified in cultures from a lymph node grown with the help of T-lymphocyte growth factor, and could apparently be propagated in adult lymphocytes and in human cord blood lymphocytes. There were some similarities between this newly recognised retrovirus and HTLV-I (Chapter Five) but there were also some differences. Not the least of these was that the Pasteur isolate appeared to kill the lymphocytes eventually, whereas HTLV-I immortalised (transformed) them. The laboratory name given to the first isolate was BRU after the patients' initials and it was to become well known. However, another Pasteur similarly identified retrovirus from a gay male with the initials LAI became even more prominent, since it later became the strain used world-wide for testing for AIDS antibodies.

A year after the Pasteur discovery, Gallo and his colleagues in the US published four papers describing the same sort of findings as those of the French workers. In the first and most well known of these papers the authors claimed to have discovered a way to grow the retrovirus in continuous culture without the cells succumbing to its supposed cytopathological effects. This was achieved by the prolonged and painstaking work on the part of Popovic, a member of the Gallo team, and involved cloning cells from an infected human cell-line (HUT-78) which eventually produced clones, including the celebrated H9 one, the cells of which were resistant to the CPE effects and enabled the cells to grow more freely. This was said to allow the growth of HIV in quantities large enough to develop a diagnostic test for AIDS.

In fact, there are several reasons for believing that this interpretation and indeed all those reached in the paper were incorrect ones, and that the Gallo group made precisely the same error that caused so much unhappiness in the early days of academic virological research, a misunderstanding that appears to have pervaded and affected a very great deal of AIDS research even up to the present day. The evidence for the belief that the resistance acquired by the cells was not to HIV but to co-cultivated mycoplasmas is considerable.

EARLY MISGIVINGS ABOUT THE ROLE OF HIV

The finding of antibodies to p24 in the serum of most of the persons with AIDS, and those presumed to be at risk of it, was interpreted in the old traditional way (Chapter Six) as being an immunological response to a hitherto unrecognised external infective agent. Since the inducing agent appeared to be the newly discovered HIV, it was claimed that it was the cause of the disease.

This, although suggestive, did not constitute proof of a causative relationship between the inducing agent and the disease, since the evolution of an 'at risk' population - by virtue of its exposure to situations involving the exchange of body fluids - enabled both opportunist and pathogenic microorganisms to propagate at a great rate, and antibodies to both types of agent - pathogenic or non-pathogenic - would be formed.

There was also the difficulty concerning the 'newness' of HIV to account for the 'new epidemic', since techniques for the isolation of retroviruses were developed and used mostly by the investigators involved in the 'War on Cancer' campaign. Until the discovery of HIV there had not been widespread interest in this narrowly specialised area, and the HIV discovery could simply have been the discovery of a hitherto unknown 'old virus'. In fact Montagnier, its discoverer, and Duesberg consider it to be an old virus. The explanation of this by Duesberg is that HIV has nothing to do with the cause of AIDS and that of Montagnier that co-factors in addition to HIV, e.g. mycoplasmas, are necessary for AIDS to occur.

Another problematical area, already mentioned in Chapter Six, is the fact that AIDS is a disease of immune-pathology and as such is likely to give rise to bizarre immunological reactions, so that standard methods used in the investigation of conventional infectious diseases are not applicable. For example, the finding of p24 sero-positivity in other similar diseases such as SLE and in chronic bacterial diseases such as leprosy - conditions in which patients are also often positive for Rheumatoid Factor (RF), which is a diagnostic marker for Rheumatoid Arthritis (RA) - opens up the possibility that this antibody may be a manifestation of immunological aberration rather than simply a straightforward response to a putative exogenous infective agent.

Papadopulos-Eleopulos *et al* (1993), a group based in Perth, Australia, have studied the AIDS problem in considerable depth, with particular emphasis on the reliability of HIV testing, especially the Western Blot test (Chapter Nine). Their basic premise has been that the failure to isolate HIV in the classic sense *i.e.* to separate the individual virions from material from other sources, especially cellular, does not allow a true validation of a diagnostic antibody test. In fact their suspicion that 'pure' HIV suspensions are contaminated by cellular materials was confirmed seven years later. This latter work, and its potential significance with respect to the aetiology of AIDS, is discussed below.

Reverting to the AIDS tests, which the Perth Group agree can be valuable if properly applied (Turner 2002), the issue is not to do with its effectiveness in the diagnosis of AIDS, it is about whether their value in this respect lies in their being one or more of the following:

a) Indicators of an HIV infection, either as the true causative agent or as a harmless accompanying virus, the presence of which serves as a surrogate marker and an AIDS risk indicator,

b) Tests for the immunological disorder that AIDS manifestly is, which are comparable with tests used for the diagnosis of Systemic Lupus Erythematosis (SLE) or Rheumatoid Arthritis (RA) as discussed in the next chapter, or

c) Indicator of infection by an episome type of agent, as also discussed in the next chapter.

TEN YEARS OF DISAPPOINTMENT

During the ten years following its launching, additional facts emerged that did not fit the orthodox

HIV=AIDS concept. It became obvious not only that HIV is not cytopathogenic *in vitro* (Chapter Two) but that it does not occur to any great extent *in vivo* either. The latter point was generally acknowledged when it was realised that the exceedingly small quantities of HIV that could be detected in the blood of patients by classical methods could not possibly account for the amount of cell destruction that occurs in advanced AIDS.

Another anomaly was that the time that elapses between sero-conversion to AIDS antibody positivity and the onset of AIDS proper, varies enormously from individual to individual, and some sero-positive persons remain healthy.

Furthermore, progress was unsatisfactory on the therapy front - the drug trials with the reverse transcriptase inhibitor zidovudine (AZT) proved to be a disappointment. They were found not to slow down the progression from asymptomatic sero-positivity to advanced AIDS as had been originally hoped, and the search for a vaccine had not produced promising results.

In fact, although successful sequencing of HIV had been claimed in France and in the US, and vast numbers of papers had been produced on various other aspects, no real progress had been made towards the development of a cure or of a prophylactic vaccine. HIV was still regarded as the causative agent of AIDS, in effect by default for want of a better solution. It had become obvious that the classical scenario that had been applicable to e.g. the development of a vaccine against poliomyelitis *i.e.* discover virus; culture it; prepare a vaccine from the concentrated virus and vaccinate the susceptible population to prevent the disease, was not going to work in the fight against AIDS.

A WATERSHED IN AIDS RESEARCH - TEN YEARS ON

By the mid-1990s matters had reached a watershed - one school of thought advocated widening the approach to the problem (Fields 1994), and the other a continuation of the thus far unproductive classic route (Wain-Hobson, Maddox 1995). The latter authors took their stance as a result of the simultaneous publication of two papers (discussed below) professing to provide a new model of viral pathogenesis purporting to explain the various anomalies.

However, even though this work introduced a supposedly 'new view' on AIDS, the simple concept actually remained intact - now immortalised in the notorious, universally known, statement by David Ho - 'It's the virus, stupid!' (Hooper 1999).

Fields - an American savant - on the other hand had pointed out that bio-medical science is not a linear pursuit and that 'sometimes answers to a problem are discovered in the most unlikely and unpredictable places. AIDS is a novel disease requiring new paradigms and a new conceptual framework regarding persistent viruses and the host response'. He advocated a widening of the narrow approach to the AIDS problem, and whilst believing that research on HIV should continue, wrote 'we must consider studies on other infectious agents and on microbial pathogenesis in general' and 'A treatment or preventive strategy for the disease is as likely to come from fundamental discoveries in fields other than AIDS research as from those targeted for AIDS.......We must give serendipity (and reasoned scientific direction) a chance to join the war on AIDS'. His concern was that by targeting too narrowly on the received wisdom on AIDS, research would risk eliminating the research project that 'holds the ultimate answers to a critical piece of the puzzle'.

He saw very clearly that even though 'our best hunches have not paid off and are not likely to do so', such was the mindset of the already established large bureaucracy and infrastructure concerned with the setting of priorities and funding of AIDS research that a change of direction would be virtually impossible to achieve. This proved to be the case and persists to this day in spite of the fact that the simple HIV equals AIDS concept is clearly not the answer to a complicated situation now of world-wide importance.

It is a curious fact that some investigators become possessive about the microorganisms they study - sometimes this is benign, as in the case of the renowned Lewis Thomas with respect to *Streptococcus* MG (1966) - but sometimes it is counter-productive, and this has particularly been the case with HIV, as evidenced by Wain-Hobson's reference (1995) to the perspicacity of 'old HIV hands' in his dismissive reference to Fields' suggestions *i.e.* 'at a time when there is discussion as how best to channel resources for AIDS research, it is worth noting that the main elements of our current picture of AIDS have come from old HIV hands, rather than from insights into other viral or microbial lifestyles'.

Such a completely unscientific attitude - the 'new view' was only an hypothesis and no other microbial life-styles had been investigated - especially one so overtly financially slanted, is indeed distressing. Premature backing from a world-renowned journal giving it a bogus stamp of authority makes it worse. In fact the 'new view' in the long run has, in reality, led to what seems to be yet another blind alley comparable to that in the pursuit of the retroviral cause of cancer, and to the introduction of potentially very dangerous therapies, which are based on demonstrably unsound premises.

THE NEW MODEL OF VIRUS PATHOGENICITY

The two papers referred to above were produced by Ho *et al* of the Aaron Diamond Institute in New York, and a team from the University of Alabama - Wei *et al.* Both groups claimed that their results provided not only an explanation of how the non-classical virus anomalies could be accommodated within the simple cause and effect scenario, but also introduced the apparently successful use of protease inhibitor drugs for the treatment of AIDS sero-positive subjects.

Although the 'new view' was strongly criticised by other workers shortly after the publications appeared, and further work published three years later virtually proved the 'new view' to be wrong, the Wei and Ho studies constituted a turning point in AIDS research. No conflicts of interest were declared as such in the *Nature* papers but it is interesting to note that several of the co-authors were based at pharmaceutical companies. Many observers would have been happier if the results had been backed at a higher level by scholars with an objective university background. The contributors based at the University of Oxford in the Wei *et al* paper were the ones who supplied the mathematical aspects but the application of mathematics to biological research particularly in the extremely complicated area of clinical medicine is notoriously difficult, and their calculations have been the object of considerable criticism.

The era of potent mixtures of powerful antiviral therapy began shortly afterwards and funding continued to be directed towards HIV almost exclusively. The hopes of a widening of the attack on

AIDS by taking into account expertise obtained in other fields of infectious disease were doomed to disappointment. The dominance of the diehard HIV=AIDS protagonists continued, the shop remained closed, and although some laboratories, such as the Garry one in New Orleans, have produced some interesting and worthwhile studies on immunological/autoimmune aspects of AIDS (discussed in Chapter Nine), the vast majority of studies have been directly or indirectly orientated in the direction of finding new therapeutic drugs and vaccines for the prevention and cure of the disease, based on the Ho and Wei models, or some variation of them.

THE 'NEW VIEW' OF AIDS AND THE ONSET OF ANTI-RETROVIRAL THERAPY

In essence, both groups in what the AIDS establishment regarded as landmark studies attempted to interfere with the balance held between what they considered to be HIV and the CD4 cells of patients by treating them with potent anti-retroviral drugs, at the same time as calculating their CD4 counts. In both sets of experiments a rapid decline in presumed viral load as measured by an RNA/PCR technique occurred, accompanied by a CD4 count increase, and it was assumed that these increases in CD4 cells numbers were equal to the number of cells that would have been destroyed but for the therapy.

The Alabama team (Wei *et al*) interpreted their results as showing that the composite lifespan of plasma virus and virus-producing cells is very short, the half-life being about two days. Moreover, they interpreted the data on the replacement of wild-type virus in plasma by the drug resistant variants, which happened after fourteen days, as indicating that HIV-viraemia is sustained mainly by a dynamic process involving continuous rounds of new virus infection and replication concomitant with rapid cell turnover.

This reading of the results was echoed by the Ho team, who claimed that 'minimum estimates of HIV production and clearance and of CD4 lymphocyte turnover indicate that replication of HIV-1 *in vitro* is continuous and highly productive, driving the rapid turnover of CD4 lymphocytes'.

The 'new view' meant that the paucity of HIV particles in the blood is a result of the virus having such stupendous killing power and the replacement of the destroyed CD4 cells is achieved so rapidly, that it is virtually imperceptible by standard methods, and that severe disease was the result of the renewal process becoming worn out.

These results and their interpretation were received with some degree of scepticism virtually immediately (HIV results in a frame - *Nature* May 1995). The main thrust of the comments was that the origin of the increases in the CD4 counts that occurred following the therapy was caused by redistribution, rather than proliferation, and several authors could see no justification for the belief that the CD4 cell counts in the disease progression towards AIDS is a consequence of their destruction by HIV (implied in the two papers) rather than a lack of production. Ascher *et al* in a particularly graphic contribution to this debate described the HIV situation proposed by the Wei/Ho groups, as 'a murder scene with far more bodies than bullets' and suggested that the fate of uninfected cells may be much more important than that of infected cells in AIDS pathogenesis. Later Wolthers *et al* (1998) produced convincing evidence, mainly in the investigation of telomere lengths, that new evidence indicated 'that CD4-cell decline cannot be explained by exhaustion of renewal due to virus induced cell destruction'. In other words, the 'new view' is incorrect. Their finding that the CD4 telomere length in CD4 cells during what is interpreted as HIV infection is close to normal implies an only slightly increased CD4 turnover in AIDS, and their overall view is that the origin of the CD4 depletion lies at the point of generation of the immune cells, perhaps due to virus attack on precursor cells, or something else, but whatever it is, 'exhaustion of renewal driven by huge turnover of CD4-T cells seems no longer a plausible cause for CD4-T-cell depletion'.

Further criticism came from Duesberg and Bialy who wrote briefly in the 'in the frame' section in *Nature* and at greater length in another publication (Duesberg and Bialy 1995) for the most part about the techniques used for measuring viral load, claiming that these gave a completely false impression and quoting previous results of some members of both teams in support of this argument.

These various concerns expressed at the time, however, did not affect the predictable launching of the new class of drugs into the clinical zone. A few months later Ho (1995) introduced the 'hit HIV, early and hard' concept for the treatment of persons infected with HIV. Part of his reasoning was based on the fact of the rapid (two weeks) appearance of resistant mutants after the initiation of therapy, mentioned above, and the rest on the new ideas of the highly dynamic nature of HIV replication in patients. He argued that 'over a typical course of HIV infection lasting about ten years, thousands of replication cycles occur, resulting in a total production of close to ten trillion virions', and that during this time unimaginable numbers of mutations arise, capable of nullifying any therapeutic measures. Thus he advocated the use of cocktails of multiple, potent, antiretroviral agents in p24-sero-positive patients as early as possible after sero-conversion. The assumption was that the earlier the treatment was started, the fewer mutants there would be and so the therapy would be more likely to have a favourable outcome.

Thus the era of the use of highly active anti-retroviral therapy (HAART) in the treatment of AIDS patients began with very high hopes of the possibility of curing the condition, but these have never been fulfilled and the whole subject has become fraught with controversy. The stages have been described in terms of the cities in which the International AIDS Conferences have been held as Berlin 1993 - doom and gloom, Vancouver 1996 - elation, Durban 2000 - waking up to the global crisis, Barcelona 2002 - the limits of success (Cohen 2002).

In brief, the treatments have been found to cause unpleasant, sometimes fatal, side-effects, and this has caused serious problems in treatment assessment, partly because of resulting patient non-compliance. The overall advice is to delay therapy as long as possible, but there is disagreement concerning what constitutes the optimal time of delay, judgement about which is based on the scale of CD4 cell depression and of the calculated viral load. Some physicians advocate giving patients 'drug holidays' or structured treatment interruptions (STIs) to provide relief from these effects, and restarting therapy when the viral load rises again, but this approach is controversial. Complications have also said to have arisen when patients present themselves having received various treatments earlier, and this makes it difficult to assess new products.

There are some reports that therapy succeeds inasmuch as acceptable CD4 counts are achieved, even though virus load has remained high, giving the impression that it is the therapy that is causing the improvement, not the presence of the virus. Thus it would seem that the therapy could be influencing the viability of other microorganisms. Also it seems likely that, as in other diseases of the immune system (Chapter Nine), relapses and remissions almost certainly happen irrespective of therapy. Various apparently successful new therapies for the treatment of rheumatoid arthritis have been tried from time to time, but in the long run results have been governed by personal factors of the patient, including placebo effects. It is also difficult to judge when claims are made for drug efficacy while additional prophylactic drug therapy is being prescribed.

Although ultimately the individual physicians and informed patients must make the decisions regarding treatment, this is not easy for either, since the drug therapy as a whole is still very much in the experimental stages and the news is not good. The therapy failures, ascribed to the apparent emergence of resistant strains brought about by haphazard use of drugs, seem to be inevitable.

BLOOD PRODUCT STUDIES

The first indication that a filterable infective agent was the cause of the AIDS epidemic was the occurrence of *Pneumocystis* pneumonia in some patients with haemophilia after treatment with the clotting agent - Factor VIII. As mentioned above (Fig. 8.1) this disease is an AIDS indicator.

Initially, in Britain at least, the preparation of Factor VIII, which involved the pooling of donor bloods, was carried out in Regional Blood Transfusion laboratories where some control of the source of the factor plasma from donors could be assured. Blood donation has always been on a voluntary basis and screening for undesirable substances has always been of the best available quality. However, in the US the factor was produced commercially in large amounts that necessarily involved very large numbers of 'donors'. Some of these were members of the American state prison population in which AIDS was quite widespread, but which were 'a good source of plasma' (Shilts 1988). Montagnier (2000) also referred to this type of problem e.g. blood supplied by drug addicts, another AIDS risk group, with blood imported from the US where there is a large blood industry. The extent of this problem was not grasped in time to prevent the exportation of the unsafe Factor VIII to Britain, France and other countries.

To all intents and purposes, the Factor VIII evidence constitutes another vast unplanned human experiment comparable to some extent with the HLA-B27 one and the ones concerning the huge increase in gay male promiscuity and drug addiction already mentioned. In the blood product situation the unintended 'experiment' consisted of the injection of large numbers of individuals with disease-producing material, the main constituent of which was derived from other human beings. The evidence seemed to point to a virological cause on the grounds that the product had been filtered, but mycoplasmas and related cell-wall-less bacteria can also pass through these filters and this was not considered at the time.

The misconception that only HIV could be the infective agent was exacerbated by Gallo and his colleagues (Blattner *et al* 1988) when they wrote 'It is noteworthy that HIV infection and not infection with any other agent is linked to blood transfusion associated AIDS' citing Peterman *et al* (1988). This statement is couched in quasi-legal jargon inasmuch as it is a carefully crafted, narrowly defined answer to a particular question, which is misleading in the overall impression conveyed. Such tactics may be acceptable as lawyer-speak but not in the language of science. For most readers of the Gallo paper, whether microbiologists or not, the impression put across by this is that Peterman *et al* made an exhaustive study of all filterable microbes that could be envisaged as being associated with blood transfusion (Chapter Three), including a search for as yet undiscovered ones, by examining a large number of bloods from patients with transfusion-associated AIDS.

In fact, Peterman *et al* only studied the transfer of blood-transfusion-acquired-p24 sero-positivity between spouses, and showed that it was transmitted in a small percentage of cases. Clearly the results in no way support the weight given to them by the Gallo group.

However the Gallo spin succeeded, and future investigators continued to believe that anti-p24 antibodies proved the presence of HIV, that HIV is the only agent that needs to be sought and the circular argument continued.

Studies claiming to prove the HIV=AIDS concept have all been at a secondary level and based on the assumption it is true.

AIDS, HIV AND HAEMOPHILIACS

Typical of these studies was one on AIDS acquired by blood transfusion (Darby *et al* 1995). These authors reported on the incidence of AIDS in 1,227 male haemophiliacs in the UK who became sero-positive for the AIDS antigen after transfusion therapy, using either Factor VIII for classical A haemophiliacs, or Factor IX for haemophilia B (Christmas Disease). The annual death rate of the sero-positive group rose steeply, regardless of the severity of the haemophilia, compared with sero-negative ones. The excess deaths were for the most part certified as due to AIDS or AIDS-related conditions.

This evidence indicates that an AIDS test performed on a patient's serum provides a satisfactory sign of AIDS or a patient at risk of AIDS resulting in this instance from the transfusion of contaminated Factor VIII. The observations made by Darby and her co-workers have no bearing on whether or not HIV causes AIDS, as the accompanying editorial claimed it to be; the HIV connection in this paper is based entirely on the belief that the connection HAD ALREADY BEEN PROVED. The fact that no other microbiological agents were looked for, either by attempts at isolation, or serological examination of patients' sera, bears this out.

The real value of this important study is that it confirms that the AIDS test is a very good indicator of the AIDS-risk status of a blood donor, and is on this count invaluable for the screening of blood before it is cleared for use.

A follow-up study on AIDS/AIDS-defining conditions occurring after treatment of patients with blood products was conducted by Sabin *et al* (1996) with the object of investigating the alternative hypothesis proposed by Duesberg, that AIDS is caused by the long-term administration of immunosuppressive foreign proteins contaminating Factor VIII, and the administration of AZT.

Patients treated with Factor VIII concentrates from 1980 -1990 were selected, and clinical events with respect to AIDS-defining diseases, CD4 lymphocytes counts, and deaths were recorded. Whereas sixteen of these events occurred in nine out of seventeen sero- positive patients, none occurred in the seventeen negative patients. The authors concluded that it was unlikely that differences in Factor VIII usage, patient age or zidovudine treatment explained the findings, and suggested that these deaths were due to HIV infection leading to progressive immune deterioration and AIDS.

As with the work of Darby *et al*, the assumption that the AIDS antibody proves the presence of HIV is based on the work of other investigators, and this study does not provide independent confirmation of the connection. The importance of this paper is the demonstration of the non-involvement of Factor VIII preparations *per se* in the aetiology of AIDS.

SIV VACCINE RESEARCH IN NON-HUMAN PRIMATES

In most investigations into human diseases of unknown aetiology it has been customary to search for an animal model, so that experiments designed to find therapies and preventive strategies, which would be unacceptable in humans, may be carried out. Chimpanzees were thought to be a potential model because of their resemblance to human beings, but repeated infusions of plasma from AIDS patients did not cause illness in the recipient animals. Although the presence of antibodies to AIDS antigens was noted in two animals, together with some degree of lymphadenopathy and immunological impairment, suggesting that the animals could provide a disease model, chimpanzees have now been abandoned as models on ethical and financial grounds.

The animals of choice for a model of human AIDS are macaque monkeys, and countless experiments have been carried out on these ill-fated creatures. The reason for this was that a disorder of immunodeficiency, sometimes with lymphomas, was found to occur in animals that were housed at some Primate Research centres in the US. This GVHD type of disorder was hastily identified retrospectively as simian AIDS and a retrovirus found in association with the disease was rubber-stamped as its cause by the same committee that named HIV as the cause of human AIDS, by naming the simian retrovirus SIV; see below. The simian immunodeficiency virus (SIV)/macaque monkey model thus became the accepted one for human AIDS and has been very widely studied in attempts to discover methods by which a vaccine for human AIDS might be developed.

This was a disaster for the macaques (Chapter Nine) made very considerably worse by the failure to apply the most obvious elementary controls in the investigations concerning vaccines, and this is discussed in the next chapter. It can be said at this point, however, that a rational interpretation of the findings, when controls were used, is that SIV does not cause simian AIDS, which is due to demonstrable laboratory manipulations, and by implication that HIV does not cause human AIDS.

In fact the general approach to vaccine research encapsulates the depressing philosophy, prevalent in AIDS research, that high technology will provide all the answers and that the past is of no importance in the haste to 'move on'. From the beginning the thinking in this area has been that cutting edge new technology involving the use of genetic engineering - e.g. a hybrid between HIV and SIV (SHIV) has been used in some studies - will solve the problems, if only the right mix can be found.

In fact, these approaches have clouded the issue considerably, and in any case the 'end-vaccines' generally speaking are ineffective. For example, Cohen discussed some of the latest vaccines in Science just before the 2002 International AIDS Conference that was held in July in Barcelona, and described e.g. the next vector in line, made by Aventis Pasteur, which primes the immune system with a live virus vector, canary pox, which carries HIV genes and then boosts it with gp 120. Rather percipiently, Cohen went on to say 'As time moves on, expect more exotic vectors such as Venezuelan equine encephalitis and unusual carrying systems such as *Salmonella* shuttling in a DNA vaccine. And if history repeats itself, you can bet that most of these vaccines will disappear before they ever make it to the finish line'.

It is not surprising that the search has been profoundly disappointing, since HIV is presumed to mutate very rapidly so that a vaccine, however ingeniously prepared, can never cover the range of variants. If, however, HIV is not the cause of AIDS as is discussed in the next chapter, quite simply the search for a vaccine is absolutely pointless.

However, it is the main object of this chapter to indicate the serious failures of control that have occurred, making much of AIDS research, including the animal studies, unreliable.

HIV AND MICROBIAL CONTAMINATION

HISTORY

The most compelling piece of evidence for mycoplasma contamination being the cause of the CPE for which HIV was blamed was provided by the Montagnier laboratory, which subsequently established unequivocally that HIV is not cytopathogenic EXCEPT IN THE PRESENCE OF CONTAMINATING MYCOPLASMAS (Chapter Two). However, the evidence was really in place from the beginning and supports this fact, and in order to develop this idea it is necessary to return to the work done in 1983 and before.

At first, Gallo and Montagnier gave different names to their virus discoveries, and were in strong disagreement for a long time concerning their classification. Gallo was convinced that the virus was an HTLV variant, even though it allegedly killed cells rather than immortalising them, whereas Montagnier regarded his BRU virus as a lentivirus. This situation was confusing, and needs to be clarified.

Accordingly an International Nomenclature Committee was convened for this purpose, which on the face of it seemed to be innocuous - normally these procedures are tedious, but without importance except to investigators who have a particular interest in the taxonomy of the organisms they are studying. This particular committee however, in what was to be a harbinger of things to come in AIDS research, went far beyond its remit of classifying the AIDS associated retroviruses , and actually effectively announced that the viruses were the causative agents of AIDS, by renaming them HIV (human immunodeficiency virus). The 'decision by committee' philosophy has been one of the worst aspects of AIDS research, for example the Durban Declaration; see below.

Before the nomenclature committee met and the issue became disputatious there had been some measure of collaboration between the Montagnier and Gallo laboratories. Cell killing was a great problem for both laboratories, each of which wanted to grow the 'new retrovirus' in quantity in order to produce sufficient to prepare materials for characterising it in various ways, including its serological and molecular properties, and, in due course, to provide a test kit for the diagnosis of AIDS.

The problem of how to grow a cytopathogenic virus for these various purposes, and in the long run to produce the promised vaccine, challenged both groups, and Montagnier was prepared to collaborate in solving this difficulty. At Gallo's request, Montagnier supplied him with cultures on two occasions.

The first sample, presented to Gallo personally by Montagnier in July 1983, consisted of supernatant fluid labelled LAV/BRU. On being told that this was not cultivable in Gallo's hands, the Paris group sent him a second specimen in September of the same year, and it was this strain, albeit labelled LAV/BRU, that was in fact the LAI strain mentioned above. In the present context the interesting point is that although the source of the strain sent to Gallo was originally unclear - for example Montagnier's associates tried to grow BRU in T-cell precursors, with inconclusive results - a 'livelier' variant appeared in the laboratory, and was eventually tracked down as being originally from patient LAI (Montagnier 2000). The crucial question at this point is the significance of the vigour of LAI, since there is no evidence that this strain was not contaminated. Indeed there is a suggestion that it was; see below.

Mycoplasmas were certainly being carried around in cultures at the time just before the Gallo papers were published, as evidenced by the heavy mycoplasma contamination of CEM cells discovered by Montagnier in cultures sent to him from the Weiss laboratory in London in February 1984 (Montagnier 2000). Later, Weiss (1991) reported that cross contaminations of HIV had almost certainly occurred between HIV cultures in his laboratory, and it seems likely, since there was no mention of mycoplasma controls, that these organisms were also at large in that laboratory. If this is the case, then work emanating from that laboratory round about that time is possibly in need of reappraisal e.g. Dalgleish *et al* (1984).

Clearly, if strict monitoring of incoming cell cultures, including their supernatants, from other laboratories, for contaminating mycoplasmas had been in force in AIDS laboratories, much of this chaos could have been avoided. Unfortunately this *sine qua non* of good laboratory practice in tissue culture technology, discussed in Chapter Two, has been overlooked, and the same admonition needs to be issued about another example of bad practice that happened in the Gallo laboratory during the work leading to the publication of the 1984 papers.

The source of the presumed mycoplasma contamination in this laboratory cannot now be known for certain, but whilst the 'vigour' of the LAI strain supplied by Montagnier gives cause for considerable concern on this score, the technique of pooling materials from various AIDS or pre-AIDS patients for inoculation into lymphoid cell-lines used by Popovic in his attempts to propagate HIV can only have exacerbated the situation. The details of this are best explained by a direct quote - 'the Gallo documents indicate, Popovic decided to pool viruses - first from three, and ultimately from ten different patients - into a single culture. The procedure has been described as 'unusual' by other researchers who point out what Popovic says is obvious - it was not a scientifically 'clean' experiment, I was trying to make a blood test........ Maybe if he dumped ten viruses into the same pot, the reverse transcriptase level would be enough to jolt one of them into action' (Culliton 1990).

This pooling technique, which could almost guarantee the isolation of mycoplasmas and indeed could have been especially improvised for the purpose, (see Montagnier and Blanchard 1993) was nevertheless used to develop the most famous cell-line for the propagation of HIV. The line - already mentioned in Chapter Two - was named H9 and celebrated as being resistant to HIV. In fact the evidence is much more in favour of the H9 cells permitting the growth of mycoplasmas or - in more logical parlance - becoming resistant to the CPE effects of the mycoplasmas (Chapter Two).

The real cause for concern about the popularity of the H9 cell-line in AIDS research is that although tissue cell-lines may become resistant to the cytopathogenic effects of contaminating mycoplasmas, the latter can still persist in a covert but viable form and are thus able to cause further errors in areas of serology, biochemistry and molecular biology.

The HUT-78 and its H9 clone have also been widely used in research on simian AIDS for the growth of SIV, and it is obvious from a perusal of the literature that similar errors of interpretation exist in that area also. (Chapter 9)

Fig. 8.2 Electron-microscopic Evidence of Resistance to Mycoplasma Contamination in the H9 cell-line

a) HIV in H9 cells (after Garry *et al* 1990 with permission from *Science*)

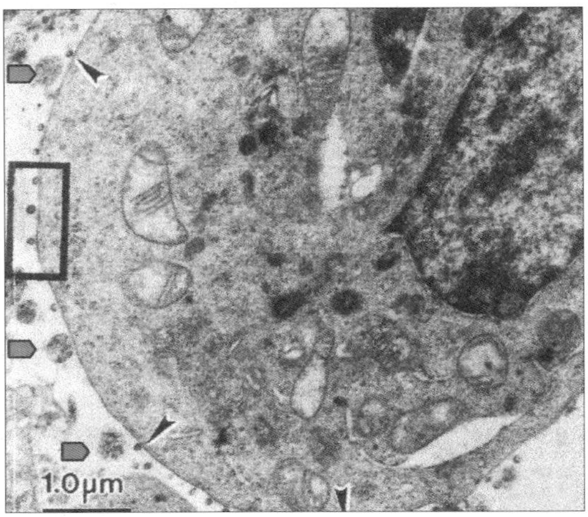

An electron-micrograph of a section of a control culture of HIV in H9 cells (clone RH9). The black arrow-heads indicate the particles believed to be HIV. The wide arrow-heads (mine) are almost certainly mycoplasma elements. Whilst it is not possible to determine the origin of these elements e.g. from the original LAI strain of HIV; from the H9 cells themselves or from materials used in processing the cultures, the preparation does demonstrate that H9 cells have acquired resistance to the CPE of mycoplasmas (Fogh *et al*, Le Maître *et al* - Chapter Two).

b) Enhanced and enlarged parts of a)

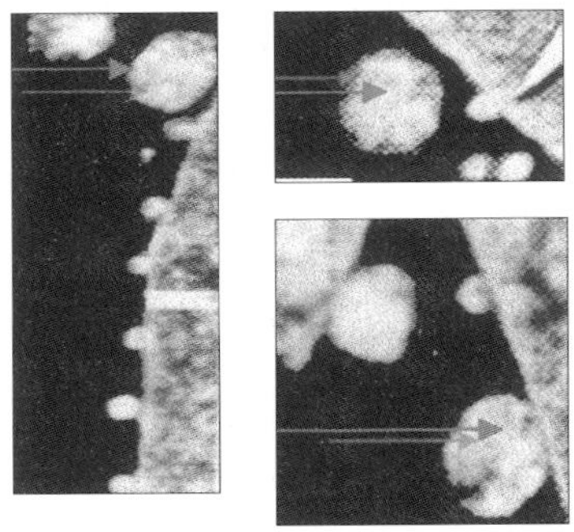

c) SIV in H9 cells

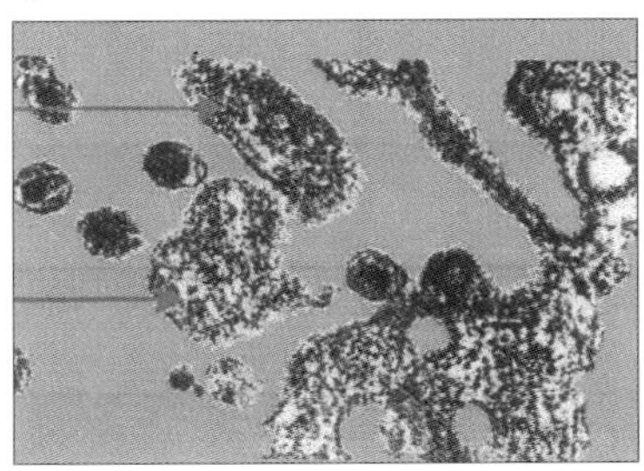

An image derived from an electron-section of SIV also grown in H9 cells (Murphey-Corb *et al* 1986) arrows (mine) indicate the putative mycoplasma contaminants

d) HTLV in MT cells

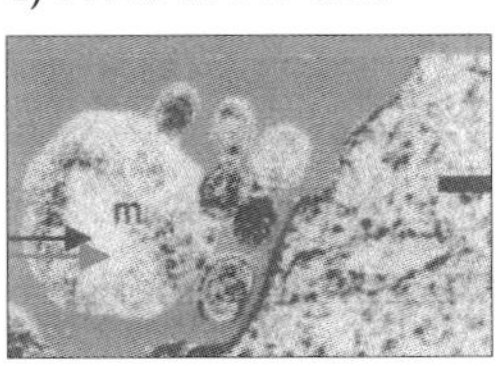

This is included for ease of size comparison of retroviral elements with mycoplasma ones (already pictured in Chapter Two - Phillips *et al* 1992)

The larger bodies in these illustrations are *circa* 300 nm in diameter, which accords well with the obsevations of Fogh *et al* (1965) who reported that the mycoplasma elements that had destroyed FL cells in culture averaged 308 nm (based on 100 measurements) - Chapter Two. The occurance of RSV particles of this size (Krishna *et al* 1998) supports the idea that retroviruses are actually cell-wall-deficient bacteria.

RETROVIRUSES AND CELLULAR CONTAMINATION

When dealing with bacteria, including mycoplasmas, which can be grown on artificial medium, contamination with other microorganisms is relatively easy to control. However, since viruses - which by definition cannot be grown in this way - need to be grown in cell-cultures, ensuring the purity of virus preparations is much more difficult. This applies not only to infective agents such as mycoplasmas, but also to the cellular materials in which they have been grown.

As previously indicated, the elementary step of electron-microscopy of retrovirus preparations for purity has been omitted since the discovery of reverse transcriptase. Reliability has been placed on physical/chemical techniques, which are greatly favoured by biochemists but which are not suitable for microbiological materials unaccompanied by microscopic methods.

Etienne de Harven (1965, 2002) has been particularly condemnatory about this failure, and his demonstration of what a pure, electron-microscopically controlled suspension of the Friend Mouse Leukaemia Virus (Fig. 8.3) looks like, explains why.

Fourteen years after the discovery of HIV and twenty seven years after the discovery of RT, the step was finally taken - two groups (Bess *et al* and Gluschankof *et al* 1997) scrutinised strains of HIV isolated using standard retrovirus isolation techniques and the results were an awful indictment of the inadequacy of the methods used in retrovirology.

Gluschankof *et al* were prompted to use electron-microscopy for the investigation of cellular contamination in their preparations of 'purified' virus, because their attempts to correlate p24 - the alleged hall-mark antigen for HIV (Chapter Nine) - with virus membrane associated HLA-DR (Chapters Six and Nine) gave erratic results, regardless of which cell-line was used. For the investigation, they studied material from standard sucrose gradients of a) HIV infected H9 cells b) PBMCs and c) non-infected H9 cells. Examination of the material prepared in the standard manner did indeed reveal a high degree of cellular contamination. In the uninfected cell preparation they found that large quantities of HLA-DR containing material banded at a density overlapping that of the 'infectious viruses'.

Electron-microscopy of the infected cell preparations showed a large population of cellular micro-vesicles ranging from 50-500 nm as compared with a minor population of virus particles of circa 100nm. Their reporting of the last figure is in line with the received information about the size of retroviruses, but on closer examination of the electro-micrographs it proves not to be accurate.

Bess *et al* published simultaneously (see Fig. 8.4) and their results are broadly in agreement with the Gluschankof group. In this case, prototype H9 cell-lines from the Gallo group (HIV-1(B) infected H9 cells, HIV-1(MN) and uninfected H9) were examined as well as uninfected cell-lines obtained from other sources.

Fig. 8.3 Electron-microscopic Control for Purity of RNA Viruses

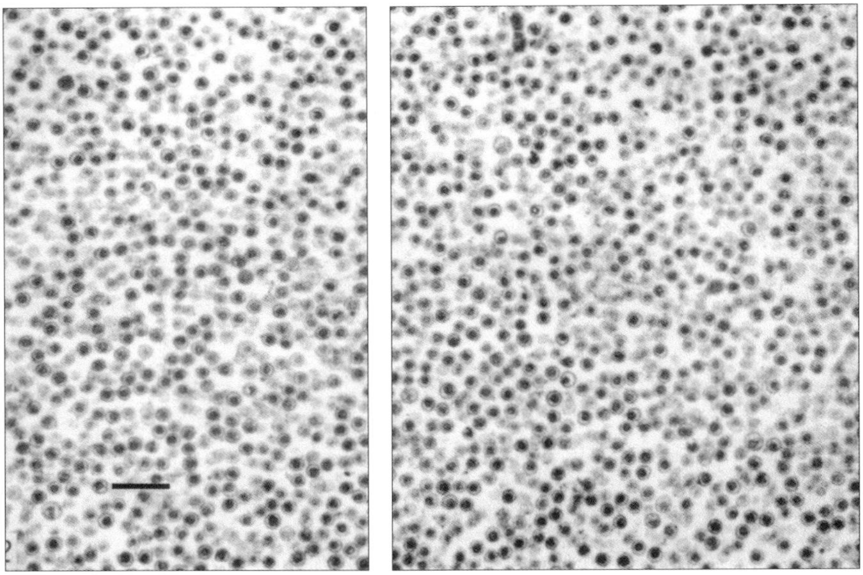

Fig. 8.3. An electronmicrograph of a preparation of the Friend leukaemia virus isolated from the plasma of leukaemic mice showing almost 100% of virus particles. Experiments designed to determine the characteristics of these viruses will be truly those of the virus *per se*. The virus preparation was made by the use of simple classic methods - blood from the mice was centrifuged to remove blood cells, filtered through 0.65μm and then 0.22μm filters and then ultracentrifuged at 30,000g followed by fixation and sectioning for electronmicroscopy using routine methods (courtesy of Etienne de Harven, first published in PathologieBiologie 1965). In complete contrast, isolation of HIV, separated from cellular components of the tissue in which is grown, has never been achieved; see 8.4.

Fig. 8.4 Electron-micrograph of Supposedly Purified HIV isolated by the Use of Standard Retroviral Techniques (Bess 2004)

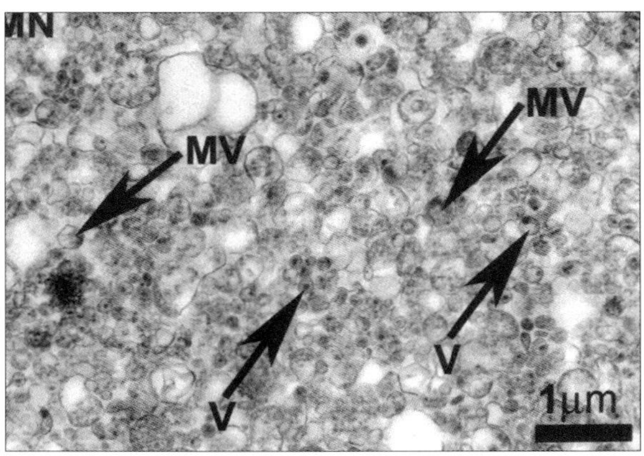

8.4 An electronmicrograph of supposedly pure HIV as prepared by standard techniques for the isolation of retroviruses employed since 1970 without the benefit of essential electronmiscopy controls. The contamination of virions with the cellular elements invalidates much of the work on retroviruses because it is impossible to determine the virus characteristics *per se* when there is so much cellular contamination. The molecular mimicry alleged to exist between HIV and human cellular proteins including HLA proteins is clearly unsound. This aspect, which casts considerable doubt on the whole concept of the alleged pathogenicity of HIV, is discussed in the next chapter with special reference to experiments on vaccine production. MV = microvesicles, V = virions.

Fig. 8.5 Sequence Homologies Claimed to Exist between HIV, Human and Mycoplasma Elements

		261	**270**
a) HIV gp 120......		VVSTQLLLNG	
Consensus HLA DR, and DQ-β chain		VVST* LI* NG	
b) HLA DR β chain	**167**	EKAGVVSTGLIQ--NGDW	**182**
HLA-DP β-chain	**165**	ETAGVVSTNLIR--NGDW	**180**
HLA-DQ β chain	**170**	ETTGVVSTPLIR--NGDW	**185**
HIV-1 gp 120	**257**	GIRPVVSTQL*L*L--NGS*L*	**272**
M. genitalium adhesin	**1224**	KLTGVVSTPL*V*N--NGQG	**1241**

Fig. 8.5 a) Sequence Young *et al* (1988), b) Sequence Bisset (1994) including a mycoplasma sequence

These sequence homologies were interpreted as indicating cross-reactivity between HIV and human cellular antigens especially HLA ones. Since the HIV particles have never been separated from the cellular elements, the simple obvious interpretation is that the presumed cross-reactivity is due to contamination of the 'pure HIV' with these elements. Thus claims that 'molecular mimicry' plays a role in HIV pathogenicity, are unfounded.

It would thus appear that the presumed HIV sequences detected by French and US groups in the mid to late 80's were composed of a mixture of elements from cells and possibly also of mycoplasma elements and this almost certainly accounts for the alleged high rate of mutations of HIV used to explain failures in the search for a vaccine and of the failure to find effective long-term therapeutic agents (see Afterword).

The purest preparation of HIV investigated by Bess *et al* was produced in MN CL4 derived from HIV-1 MN, which had undergone rigorous purification processes resulting in the occurrence of proportionally more virus-like particles. The interesting point here is the fact that an increase in the numbers of particles seems to correlate with an increase in p24 production, and the possible significance of this is discussed in the next chapter. In fact, these particles show more variation in size, more in accordance with the observations of others using more precise EM measurements, and some are indistinguishable from particles of bacterial sub-cellular-elements (see below).

RETROVIRUSES IN RETROSPECT

BACK TO THE FUTURE

Although in this case the retrovirus was HIV, the same methods had been used to isolate and characterise retroviruses from the beginning, and the implication is that until 1997 retrovirus work was performed by investigators who lacked understanding of the materials they were handling, and this of course goes hand in hand with potential disasters in interpretations. In fact, this calls for a return to the drawing board - effectively a return to 1970, *i.e.* the Temin and Baltimore papers announcing the discovery of RT (Chapter Five).

In the Baltimore paper the R-MLV was virus obtained from plasma of infected Swiss mice by 'differential centrifugation' in the first place, and thereafter by further centrifugation and re-suspension. His RSV preparation was the Prague strain and was 'purified from tissue culture fluid by 'differential centrifugation'. No mention was made of checking for either bacterial or cellular contamination by electron-microscopy to ensure virus purity.

The RSV strain examined by Temin, probably the Bryan strain, was derived from chicken cells in culture. Although received opinion is that the RT that was demonstrated came unequivocally from the virions in each case, Baltimore in his introduction, although not in his conclusions, mentioned the possibility that the RNA tumour viruses could 'induce the synthesis soon after infection' as opposed to the idea that the viruses could 'carry the enzyme into the cell as part of the virion'.

Some investigators believe that this is the true explanation, because of the fact that retroviruses totally free of cellular material have never been obtained, and in some 'pure virus' preparations the virus-like particles are so extremely scarce that it seems certain that most, or all of the activity, including RT, comes from the cellular debris and not from the virus particles (Chapter Five). This is discussed further in Chapter Nine.

THE CASE FOR RETROVIRUSES BEING SUB-CELLULAR ELEMENTS OF BACTERIA

Since RSV was discovered to be a filterable cancer-causing agent it has been assumed to be a virus, although it is now widely recognised that smaller elements of bacteria including mycoplasmas are not excluded by this type of filtration. I have already explained that in the past such filterable forms have been identified as viruses until they have been recognised as bacteria *i.e.* mycoplasmas, by virtue of their ability to in grow cell-free medium.

In the case of RSV, there has been a little known apparently successful attempt to grow it on artificial medium (Alexander-Jackson 1970). This investigation was based on the need to determine the true nature of the viruses hitherto known as RNA tumour viruses in view of the then recent realisation that a DNA phase was a necessary part of their life-cycle (Chapter Five). The work that had particularly attracted Alexander-Jackson's attention to this was that of Force and Stewart (1964), who had demonstrated that the growth and transforming ability of RSV can be prevented by DNA antagonists such as 5 iodo-2 desoxyuridine. She pursued this aspect using an ultraviolet spectrogramic microscope and was able to follow RNA and DNA activities in parallel with the cultural experiments and electron-microscopy.

Academic virology was in its infancy, in the sixties and early seventies, and ideas concerning the structure of viruses were relatively new, but the technology to verify such viewpoints was not then widely available. With the advent of computer graphics a spurious authority was lent to images of retroviruses based on the well-established structures of the other viruses such as that of the Herpes group. HIV has been the subject of a great deal of this sort of treatment and the images produced as a result of these pre-conceived ideas have proved to be very convincing and have given the impression that they are accurate representations. Recent work has shown that these depictions are not accurate and have shown that RSV and HIV are not icosohedral nor are their particles of uniform size as presupposed by retrovirologists in the 1970s. The particles *per se* in fact closely resemble CWDs with respect to the variation in the sizes of the smaller CWDs and their morphology.

Fig. 8.6 Electron Sections of Particles Identified as HIV Compared with CWD-forms of Bacteria

a)

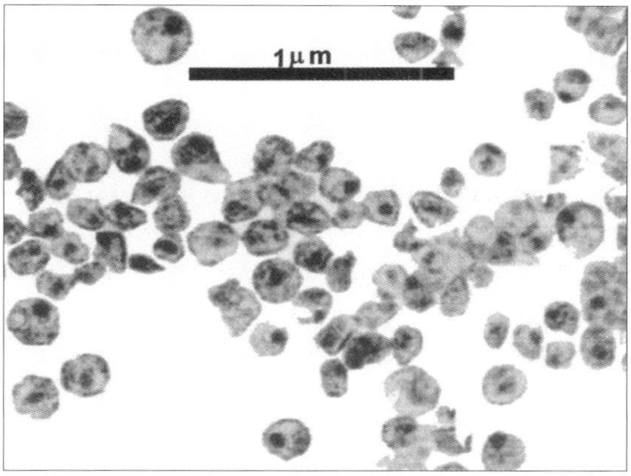

a) This is an adaption of the image of the rigorously 'purified' MNCL 4 preparation of HIV with the microvesicle particles eliminated. The bar, which was inaccurate in the original Bess *et al* has been corrected (see below),

b)

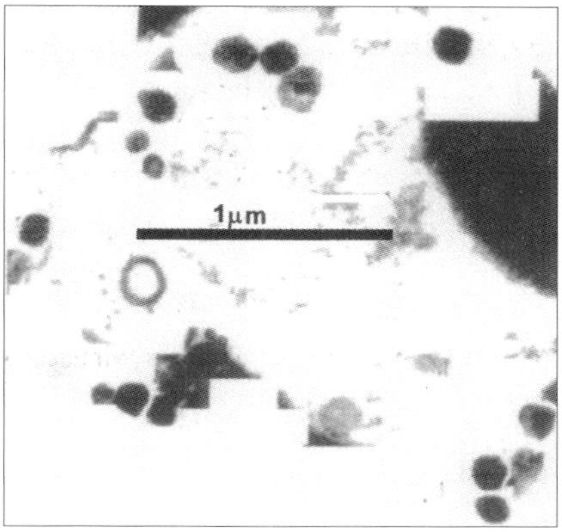

b) An electron-section of a 'Large Body' of *Yersinia enterocolitica* (already mentioned in Chapter One). The particles fall into the size-range of retroviruses (see below). Montagnier remarked on the similarity when I visited his laboratory in 1992.

I am very much indebted to Julian Bess (2004) for explaining to me that the intention of the Bess *et al* (1997) publication was simply to show that 'pure' HIV preparations are contaminated with cellular components derived from the tissue-cells. In the course of their preparations an error occurred with regard to the bar-size, which did not detract from the intention to demonstrate cellular contamination of 'pure' HIV preparation but was of critical importance to interested microbiologists. In fact, the original bar was 66% of what it should have been. With the help of the electron-microscopist - Mr. Kunio Nagishima - I have been supplied with new images from the same original preparations and have been able to estimate the size-range of the presumed HIV particles.

Examination of 150 particles revealed a size-range between 70nm - 225nm. This places them well within the size-range of bacterial CWD forms (Fig.8.6b and Chapter Two).

Krishna *et al* (1998) interpreted the range of particle sizes (70nm-370nm) they found in RSV as being due to mutations of the virus. The larger forms could easily be confused with the bigger CWD elements of bacteria. If these forms are in fact CWD forms rather than retroviruses it could be that larger elements, including elements by which they could be identified, are lost during the 'purification' proess, resulting in the concentrtion of the smaller retrovirus-like forms (compare mycoplasmas Chapter Two).

In the next chapter, the way in which these particles, if indeed they are of bacterial origin, could function as vectors of human DNA in the human immunopathologies is discussed.

SUMMARY AND CONCLUSIONS

A background to the AIDS problem is provided, from the first recognition of the epidemic and the discovery of HIV and the p24 antibody, through to the Ho *et al* and Wei *et al* views of the mechanism of AIDS pathogenicity and the development of HAART therapy. AIDS and studies on haemophiliacs are discussed and it is pointed out that these are undermined by the failure to investigate the possibility that other microorganisms such as haemoplasmas might be involved. It is indicated that failure to ensure freedom of HIV from cellular materials derived from tissue cultures also means that many of the basic notions underlying the HIV equals AIDS are faulty. Finally it is tentatively suggested that the retroviruses involved in some clonal disorders, including AIDS, may be sub-cellular forms of bacteria.

REFERENCES

Barre-Sinoussi J.C., Chermann J.C., Rey F. *et al* (1983) Isolation of a T-Lymphocyte Retrovirus from a Patient at risk for Acquired Immune Deficiency Syndrome (AIDS)
Science 220 868-871

Bess, J.W., Gorelick, R.J. Bosche, W.J. *et al* (1997) Microvesicles are a Source of Contaminating Cellular Proteins found in Purified HIV-1 Preparations
Virology 230 134-144

Bisset, L (1992) The *Mycoplasma genitalium* Adhesin Protein and Several Human Class 11 MHC Proteins Exhibit Sequence Homology: Possible Ramifications for the Development of Autoimmunity
Autoimmunity 14 167-168

Bisset, L (1994) Molecular Mimicry in the Pathogenesis of AIDS: The HIV/MHC/Mycoplasma triangle
Medical Hypotheses 43 388-396

Blattner W., Gallo R.C. and Temin H.M. (1988) HIV Causes AIDS
Science 241 514-517 (Policy Forum)

Buttrey, T.V. (1994) Calculating Ancient Coin Production 11: Why it cannot be done
The Numismatic Chronicle 150 351

Cohen J. (2002) Confronting the Limits of Success
Science 296 2320-2324

Culliton B. (1990) Inside the Gallo Probe
Science 248 1494-1498

Dalgleish, A. G., Beverley, P.C.L. Clapham, P.R. *et al* (1984) The CD4 (T4) antigen is an essential component of the receptor for the AIDS retrovirus
Nature 312 763-765

Darby, S.C., Ewart, D.W. and Giangrande, P.L.F. (1995) Mortality before and after HIV infection in the complete U.K. population of haemophiliacs
Nature 377 79-82

de Harven, E (1965) - Fig. 8.3

de Harven (2000) pers comm

Duesberg, P.H. (1987) Retroviruses as Carcinogens. Expectations and Reality
Perspectives in Cancer Research 47 1199-1220

Duesberg, P. (1988) HIV is Not the Cause of AIDS
Science 241 514-517 (Policy Forum)

Duesberg, P. (1995) Inventing the AIDS Virus
Regnery Publishing, Inc. Washington, D. C.

Duesberg, P. and Bialy, H. (1996) Responding to 'Duesberg and the new view of HIV'
Kluwer Academic Publishers. Printed in the Netherlands

Fields B. N. (1994) AIDS: time to turn to basic science
Nature 369 95-96

Garry, R.F., Fermin, C.D., Hart, D.J. *et al* (1990) Detection of a Human Intracisternal A-Type Retroviral Particle Antigenically Related to HIV
Science 250 1127-1129

Gluschankof, P., Mondor, I., Gelderblom, H.R. *et al* (1997) Cell Membrane Vesicles are a major contaminant of gradient enriched Human Immunodeficiency Virus type-1 Preparations
Virology 230 125-133

HIV results in a frame (1995)
Nature 375 193-198

Ho D. D, Avidan U, Perelson A. S. *et al* (1995) Rapid turnover of plasma virions and CD4 lymphocytes in HIV-1 infection
Nature 373 123-126

Ho D.D. (1995) Time to hit early and hard
New Eng. J Med 333 450-451

Hooper, E. (1999) The River
Allen Lane The Penguin Press

Krishna, N.K., Campbell, S., Vogt, V. *et al* (1998) Genetic Determinants of Rous Sarcoma Virus Particle Size
J Virol. 72 564-577

Maddox J. (1995) Duesberg and the new view of HIV
Nature 373 189

Montagnier, L. and Blanchard, A (1993) Mycoplasmas as Cofactors in Infection Due to the Human Deficiency Virus
Clinical Infectious Diseases 17 309-315

Montagnier, L. (2000) 'virus'
W.W. Norton & Company New York London

Mullis, K.B. (1995) Foreward to Duesberg's book, 'Inventing the AIDS Virus'
Regency Publishing, Inc. Washington D.C.

Papadopulos-Eleopulos, E., Turner, V.F. and Papadimitriou, J.M. (1993) Is Western Blot Proof of HIV Infection?
Bio/tech 11 697-707

Peterman, T.A., Stoneburner, R.L. Allen, J.R. *et al* (1988) Risk of human immunodeficiency virus transmission from heterosexual adults with transfusion associated infections.
J. Am. Med .Assoc 259 55

Sabin, C.A., Pasi, K.J. and Philips, A.N. (1996) Comparison of immunodeficiency and AIDS defining conditions in the HIV negative and HIV positive men with haemophilia A
B.Med J 312 207-209

Shilts, R. (1988) And the Band Played on
Penguin Books USA Inc.

Thomas, Lewis (1966)* see below

Turner, V.T. (2002) pers. comm.

Wain-Hobson S. (1995) Virological mayhem
Nature 373 102

Wei X, Ghosh S. K, Taylor M. E. *et al* (1995) Viral dynamics in human immunodeficiency virus type 1 infection
Nature 373 117-123

Weiss R. (1991) Provenance of HIV strains
Nature 349 374

Wolthers, K.C., Schuitemaker, H. ad Miedema, F. (1998) Rapid CD4 T-cell turnover in HIV-1 infection: a paradigm revisited
Immunology Today 19 45-48

Young, J.A.T. (1988) HIV and HLA similarity
Nature 333 215

** Lewis Thomas visited my laboratory around this time and told me he had an 'avuncular affection' for Streptococcus MG. He also said that he had a hunch that L-forms were involved in RA.*

Note added in proof - The work of the Perth group including the paper on MCT transmission and a recent one 'A critique of the Montagnier evidence for the HIV/AIDS hypothesis (2004) can be found on www.theperthgroup.com.

Weiss, R., Wain-Hobson, S. The Durban Declaration.
Nature 2000 406 15-16

Stewart, G.T. et al. Not all accept the Durban Declaration.
Nature 2000 407 286

CHAPTER NINE

AIDS AND THE OTHER IMMUNOPATHOLOGIES

'Multifactorial is multignorance. Most factors go away when we learn the real cause of disease.'

Lewis Thomas (1992)

'The most likely interpretation of SLE is that, for some reason basically genetic, forbidden clones appear which can react with a wide variety of body components. This must open the way for what may be quite legitimately referred to as a chronic civil war within the body.'

Burnet (1962)

'Thus, in place of the hypothetical somatic mutation of the antibodies (clones) I would substitute a quasi mutation of the body's own antigens as the extreme case of an infective aetiology of immune pathogenesis.'

Pease (1965)

'It should be noted that such experiments (Walter Reed's ones on the transmission of Yellow Fever with human volunteers) are not permitted today, and accordingly it is exceedingly difficult to establish whether a newly isolated virus is the cause of a disease or merely a fellow traveller with the undiscovered etiologic agent.'

Ginsberg (1980)

GENERAL INTRODUCTION 139

THE AS/HLA-B27 CONNECTION 141

MOLECULAR MIMICRY (MM) AND TRANSIENT ARTHROPATHIES - THE POSSIBLE ROLE OF CWD FORMS 142

EPISOMES IN AS 143

GVHD AND AIDS 143

THE SIGNIFICANCE OF THE CLASSIC AIDS PROTEIN (P24) 144

continued overleaf

contents continued

ANTI-P24 IN OTHER GVHD-LIKE IMMUNOPATHOLOGIES 147

MOUSE MODELS 147

HUMAN TRANSPLANTATION AND P24 148

SIMIAN AIDS AND VACCINES 149

LABORATORY HISTORY OF THE DAVIS MACAQUES 151

VACCINE STUDIES INDICATING THAT SIV DOES NOT CAUSE SIMIAN 'AIDS' 152

CONFIRMATION OF THE STOTT RESEARCH 153

GVHD - THE MODUS OPERANDI OF AIDS AND OTHER IMMUNOPATHOLOGIES 155

MICROCHIMERISM, GVHD AND ALLO-IMMUNITY 156

THE TRANSMISSION OF AIDS 157

P24 AND THE PROPOSED AIDS EPISOME COMPOSITION 157

SUMMARY 158

GENERAL INTRODUCTION

Before the onset of the AIDS epidemic, a group of disorders of the immune system, in which the seemingly normal cells of the body are attacked by the body's own immunological defence mechanisms, had been recognised and investigated for over a century. Generally speaking, these conditions are called autoimmune, which is a useful, but rather vague, definition. This imprecision is a reflection of the fact that the aetiology of the disorders is not understood.

The damage inflicted in these conditions ranges from mild to very serious and sometimes even life-threatening and may be confined to a single organ, e.g. thyroiditis; to several organs and tissues or be systemic e.g. Systemic Lupus Erythematosis (SLE). This latter disorder is not as common or as well known as Rheumatoid Arthritis (RA), another autoimmune condition, but it manifests so many classic symptoms of the disorders that it is regarded by many investigators as the autoimmune disease *par excellence*. It resembles AIDS in many attributes, particularly with respect to autoantibody production, (Table 9.1)and in about a third of cases there is evidence of p24 - the classic AIDS antigen - but so far no causative microbial agent has been satisfactorily demonstrated.

Table 9.1 Autoantibodies Detected in AIDS Patients

Auto-antibody specificity	Associated clinical condition
Lymphocyte antigens	Lymphocytopaenia
Platelet antigen/s	Thrombocytopaenia
Neutrophil antigens	Neutropenia
Erythrocyte antigens	Anaemia
Nerve antigens	Peripheral neuropathy
Brain antigens	Cognitive disorders
Sperm seminal plasma antigens	Infertility
Nuclear antigens (ANA, histones DNA etc.)	Autoimmunity, auto-immune complexes
Collagen	Arthropathies
Thymic hormone	Immune disorders
Thyroglobulin	Thyroid disease
Immunoglobulin	Immune dysregulation
HLA class I class II	Immune complexes

Over the years numerous attempts have been made to identify causative agents for the disorders, especially for RA, and the literature on the subject is very extensive, and innumerable meetings have been held about it, but the upshot is that there is no convincing evidence that classic infective agents are aetiologically associated with these disorders. Currently, endogenous retroviruses are in fashion as potential aetiological agents (Chapter Five).

This lack of definitive infective agents has meant that classification of the disorders is excessively difficult, and reliance has to be placed on a variety of clinical observations and laboratory tests. Diagnosis often involves the use of non-specific tests such as the detection of Rheumatoid Factor (RF), and/or anti-nuclear antibodies (ANA) and such tests as Erythrocyte Sedimentation Rates (ESR); see Appendix 1.

The general features, clinical and laboratory, of autoimmune disease, particularly those grouped as collagen ones, are shared in varying proportions between the members of the group, with a considerable degree of overlap from one named disease to another. The properties associated with the conditions that are regarded as classic autoimmune diseases are; serological irregularities, including the occurrence of autoantibodies; a tendency to respond to treatment with corticosteroids and other drugs that suppress immunological responses; a progressive course, sometimes slow, sometimes rapid, but often variable, with improvements - not necessarily as a result of therapy - and relapses.

It was recognised early on by many practitioners that the diseases in question, in addition to having a frustratingly elusive infective element, also 'ran in families' - that somehow there was a genetic element involved. The discovery of the HLA-B27/Ankylosing Spondylitis connection (Chapter Six) clarified and confirmed this concept.

The HLA-B27/AS association and the discovery of other similar, albeit not so strong, HLA/disease connections, e.g. certain Class II DR ones with RA and AIDS, are clearly of critical importance, since the histocompatability/self antigens lie at the core of the immune system and, thereby, at that of the disordered immune system. However, in spite of the recognition of this fact, there is still no widely accepted concept that accommodates the true significance of the connection.

One very widely explored avenue has been the molecular mimicry one, already mentioned in Chapter Six. The idea that a micro-organism contains antigen that mimics a body component, so that the immunological system is stimulated to produce antibodies that react, not only with the invading organism, but also with body components thus damaging them, is at first sight an attractive one. It is most compelling in the case of the HLA-B27 connection. However, this simple explanation fails to explain why only a small proportion of HLA-B27 individuals have AS in spite of the fact that all such individuals are exposed to the cross-reacting bacteria.

The laboratory test for HLA-B27 positivity is an invaluable diagnostic aid for the confirmation of a diagnosis of AS, but only when it is taken into consideration with clinical observations; taken alone it is of very little significance except as being a very slight indication of being marginally 'at risk' of AS.

(It is important to note that this has only a very superficial resemblance to the AIDS test, which is discussed later.)

As far as being a factor in the disease, however, there is no doubt that there must obviously be other factors involved. The NGE concept originally presented as the episome theory of autoimmune disease (Pease 1965) provides the missing factor in the form of alien DNA colonisation of the nuclei of patients' body cells, in a manner parallel to that proposed for the aetiology of the malignancies (Chapter Seven). In the case of these immunological disorders it is proposed that the colonising DNA interferes with the MHC/HLA related DNA that undermines the function of the immune system, as opposed to the function of the system of growth regulation in the malignancies.

The current perception of these diseases is that they are of clonal origin, and this is in accordance with the original views of Burnet and his concept of the aetiological significance of the emergence of 'forbidden clones', proliferating and causing havoc with the immunological defence processes of the patient.

However, whereas Burnet believed that the 'forbidden clones' arose from within the patient, present day information is more in accord with the his GVHD model (Chapter Six), in which the undesirable clones are of alien, not endogenous origin, which makes them allo-immunities rather than autoimmunities. Certain clinical conditions - the so-called collagen diseases such as Sjogren's Syndrome (SS), SLE and primary biliary cirrhosis (PBC) have a remarkable resemblance to GVHD, and patients contract the disorders naturally, i.e. without therapeutic interventions or undue exposure to parenteral procedures. The cases that are associated with such interventions are those GVHDs that occur after therapeutic transplantation procedures. The considerable resemblance between AIDS and GVHD was noted even before HIV was discovered, but this possible *modus operandi* for AIDS causation became over-shadowed with the identification of HIV as the causative agent.

Support for the idea of a GVHD origin of some auto-allo immune diseases has come recently, from newly emerging studies on maternal and foetal cell-trafficking (micro-chimerism), which represents a natural mechanism for the acquirement of alien lymphocytes by both mother and foetus. The possibility of GVHD/allo immune diseases e.g. SS and SLE being mediated by this route is currently being studied by several laboratories.

It is the purpose of this chapter to present an up-dated version of the episome theory of the classic immunopathologies, with special emphasis on the possibility that AIDS may fall into this category of disease rather than being a conventional viral infection. The term I originally used for the putative infective DNA was episome, Jacob and Wollman (Chapter One). Since then, the terms episome and plasmid have come to overlap to some extent, with plasmids originally referring to bacterial DNA separate from the main nuclear body, and episome referring to plasmids capable of existing autonomously or integrated into the main nucleus. Here I propose to use the terms interchangeably as the context demands.

THE AS/HLA-B27 CONNECTION

The discovery of this relationship marked the beginning of an era, inasmuch as it pinpointed the fact that there is a definite connection between a 'self' antigen and a group of diseases - the most outstanding one being AS - and thus paved the way to an understanding that self/HLA antigens are of critical importance in diseases involving the immune system. However, the precise nature of the connection still remains something of a mystery, and it is the purpose of this section to explain the molecular mimicry aspect, and to introduce the episome concept of the immunopathologies.

The diseases that are connected with HLA-B27 include AS, Crohn's Disease, Reiter's Syndrome and the reactive arthritis following infection of HLA-B27 subjects with gram-negative bacteria such as *Yersinia*, *Shigella*, *Campylobacter*, and *Salmonella*. They are sometimes referred to as the sero-negative (for RF) arthropathies and the discovery of the HLA-B27 connection has added another useful classification marker.

The HLA-B27 and bacterial disease connections led Alan Ebringer and his colleagues (King's College, London UK) to investigate the possibility that molecular mimicry is involved in the pathogenesis of AS, in the way comparable to that widely quoted as happening in RF with respect to streptococci (Chapter Six). The group found cross-reactivity between *Klebsiella* and HLA-B27 by using a variety of techniques, and several other groups, including our laboratory, attempted to reproduce these results, not always successfully, although this may have been due to the use of varying techniques.

The most important point to note in this work is that whilst the Ebringer group found cross-reactivity between bacteria and lymphocytes from HLA-B27 subjects, irrespective of the presence of AS, our group and the Geczy group found that the cross-reactivity happened only with lymphocytes from patients with AS. The implication of the latter results is that AS lymphocytes are different from the normal ones. Further work in our laboratory, demonstrated by the use of ELISA as well as haemagglutination techniques, gave similar results with lymphocytes from patients with CD (Pease *et al* 1980, 1986).

We found also that a difference between normal and diseased lymphocytes could be detected by the fact that in standard lymphocytotoxicity tests only the latter were lysed in the presence of some normal rabbit sera (MacKintosh and Pease 1982). This suggests that the diseased lymphocytes have a degree of fragility possibly analogous to that of CD4 lymphocytes in AIDS patients that seem 'primed to die' (Montagnier 2000). This latter situation seems to be related to GVHD, which appears to be a major factor in immunological disease; see below.

MOLECULAR MIMICRY (MM) AND TRANSIENT ARTHROPATHIES - THE POSSIBLE ROLE OF CWD-FORMS

The MM demonstrated by the Ebringer group between gram-negative bacteria and HLA-B27 suggests that the immunological system has some difficulty in distinguishing between 'self' and the infecting bacterium, and since the CWD forms of bacteria have a predilection for joints, this could be the explanation for the post bacterial arthritis when this is transitory or even prolonged. In the case of diseases associated with HLA, the molecular mimicry rendering the bacteria less easy to recognise as foreign could be the explanation of the arthritic and other effects of relatively short duration that sometimes follow infection with a variety of gram-negative bacteria.

EPISOMES IN AS

The model for this is shown in Fig 9.1, which shows a bacterium containing DNA material in the form of a plasmid /episome which is transported into a human lymphocyte, possibly via a CWD form of the bacterium. In accordance with the theory, discussed at greater length below, it seems likely that the episome would contain coding for part of the HLA-B27 protein.

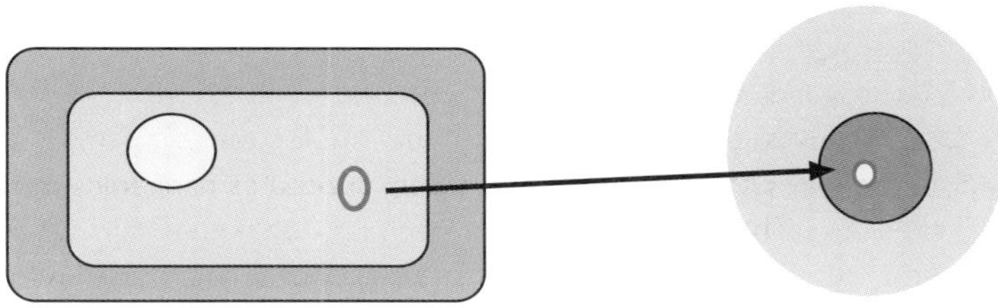

Fig. 9. 1 Infection of lymphocytes with foreign DNA coding for alloantigens would set up a situation in which two sets of lymphocytes are present with the potential of attacking one another. Some pointers to this are evident in the predispositions of certain tissue types (HLAs) being associated with particular autoimmune diseases. In the case of the connection between HLA-B27 and AS it seems likely that the putative episome/plasmid would encode for a recognisable fragment of HLA-B27, which *would* facilitate the entry of the DNA because of the random mimicry effect Evidence for the existence of a plasmid in the aetiology of AS was produced by Geczy *et al*, who believed it to be connected with a transforming factor concerned with the change from AS to AS+ lymphocytes.

The observations from the Geczy laboratory and our own indicate that there are several possible gram-negative putative bacterial hosts capable of harbouring the relevant DNA sequences.

GVHD AND AIDS

The striking resemblances between GVHD and AIDS were reported by Shearer in 1983 and since then more evidence in support of this concept has been forthcoming. Habeshaw and Dalgleish (1989) compared the immunodeficiency in AIDS with the chronic allogenic and semi-allogenic GVHD in mouse models, and reported that the clinical characteristics of these mice, such as wasting, gut infection, lymphoid depletion, opportunist infections and skin rashes are 'clinically not unlike those seen in ARC/AIDS patients'. Dalgleish (1992) wrote further about the GVHD approach and produced a list of the similarities between AIDS and GVHD in both clinical and laboratory tests (Table 9.2).

Clearly, had HIV not been discovered and named as the cause of AIDS, this perspective would have received considerably more attention. As matters stand, a number of observations have been made in animal studies, especially in the simian model of human AIDS that strongly suggest that AIDS is a GVHD and that both HIV and SIV are not the aetiological agents. In other words, the test that is diagnostic for AIDS or pre-AIDS is not a test for HIV. In order to pursue this idea it is necessary to discuss AIDS testing and the definitive AIDS protein in detail.

Table 9.2 Similarities between AIDS and GVHD

Opportunist Infections
Lymphomas
Lymphadenopathy,
Change in CD-8 total and Relative Number
Suppressor Cells selective for CD-4 Cells
Skin Lesions
Increased Cytokine Production
Cytotoxicity for Autologous Cells
Cytotoxicity for allo-antigens
B cell hyper-reactivity
Gastro-intestinal Symptoms/illness
AIDS Defining Antibody p24*
AIDS gp- 120 antibody occurs*

Starred items are my additions (to those of Dalgleish 1992). These antibodies occur in allo-immune/GVHD mice (Kion and Hoffman - Fig. 9.4). Effectively the allo-immune mice would be diagnosed as HIV sero-positive. This suggests that the AIDS tests (Figs. 9.2 and 9.3) are really tests for auto and allo antibodies, which have nothing to do with the external agent - HIV.

Experiments concerning the protection from 'simian AIDS' by vaccines have shown that macaque monkeys are protected from the disease, by vaccines consisting of cellular antigens only, irrespective of whether the HIV homologue - the simian immunodeficiency virus (SIV) - is present, supporting the view that retroviruses are irrelevant in both human and simian AIDS.

THE SIGNIFICANCE OF THE CLASSIC AIDS PROTEIN (P24)

It has been pointed out in previous chapters that the main AIDS antibody - p24 antibody - was first discovered by the Montagnier group in a patient at risk from AIDS in 1983. Since that time AIDS testing has been refined, and many sources of the initially high level of false sero-positivity that resulted in erroneous diagnoses have been eliminated. The two main AIDS tests are shown in Figs 9.2 and 9.3.

Detection of this antibody in an individual is a good indication that an individual either has AIDS or is at risk of AIDS, provided due regard is taken of clinical and other laboratory tests, such as CD-4 count, and of his or her life-style. Although sexual promiscuity has been emphasised as a risk factor in the patient's life-style, with the attendant emphasis on the use of condoms, the risk of therapeutic procedures involving substandard medical interventions such as the re-use of unsterilised disposable hypodermic syringes has probably been greatly underestimated. Due note of this possibility must be taken in assessment of risk. In addition to AIDS diagnosis, the detection of sero-positivity for p24 is an essential part of the screening of blood supplies for therapeutic use. It is a method of selection of AIDS risk donors, and no doubt in the process pathogenic agents associated with AIDS will also be screened out.

However, as already intimated, the presence of an anti-p24 antibody does not necessarily mean that the antibody *per se* is elicited by a specific external microbiological agent. This classic immunological response to an infective agent such as *Salmonella typhi* is not easily applicable to diseases of the immune system itself, because in this type of disorder antibody responses are aberrant by definition. Autoantibodies are by definition very common in the diseases of immunopathology, and in AIDS they occur in abundance (Table 9.3) and as will be discussed below, there is evidence that the p24 antibody is also an autoantibody to a widely-conserved cellular one. It is of vital importance to discover the true nature of this antigen *i.e.* whether it is of external or endogenous origin, since this must affect the approaches to therapy and prevention. If the antigen is purely of a cellular nature then it is obvious that vaccines in the normal sense would be ruled out of the question.

The origin of the p24 antibody in the individuals concerned could be a self-limiting condition as opposed to a sign of inevitable progression to advanced AIDS. This effect can be reproduced in the laboratory by injecting animals with species homologous antigens (allo-antigens). Various autoantibodies are elicited but these are normally self-limiting and harmless.

The human equivalent to this could be a mild GVH (Chapter Five) effect resulting in the production of p24 antibodies in the humans in continuous acts of anal sex where injected allo antigens could escape into the blood stream of the recipient (Chapter Eight). These antibodies can remain in the serum for months or even years and it is of very great importance to ascertain that the sero-positivity has been taken in the context of the clinical condition of the patient, as already mentioned, before a diagnosis of AIDS is made. It is now recognised that many individuals have the 'AIDS' antibody but do not develop AIDS.

This non-progression to AIDS is attributed to various drug regimes that have been developed since AZT as discussed in the last chapter. The possibility of health care being a factor in the spread of AIDS is discussed in the Afterword.

Fig. 9.2 Elisa testing for the p24 'AIDS Antibody' (After Williams et *al* 1989)

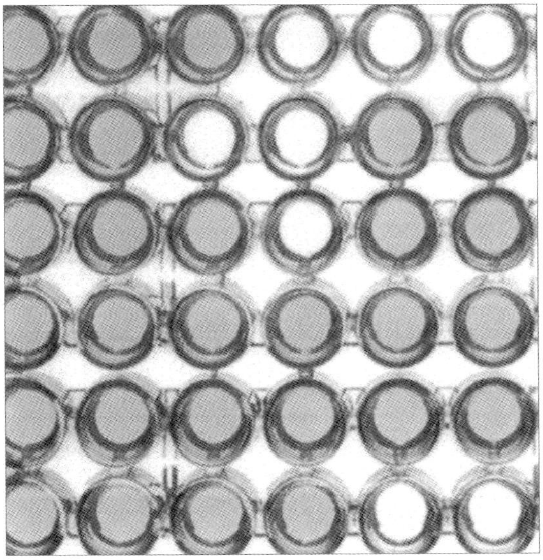

Fig. 9.2 Enzyme-linked immunosorbent assay (ELISA). The patient's serum is added to p24 antigen, which has been bound first to the well of a micro-titre plate. If the corresponding antibody is present the serum will become attached to the bound antigen and can be detected by the addition of anti-human serum coupled to an enzyme such as horse radish peroxidase, which converts to a coloured end product (yellow in this example - see colour image after page 111). Optical scanning is used to determine the extent of antigen presence.

Fig. 9.3 Western Blot (WB) Test for Antibodies Diagnostic for AIDS

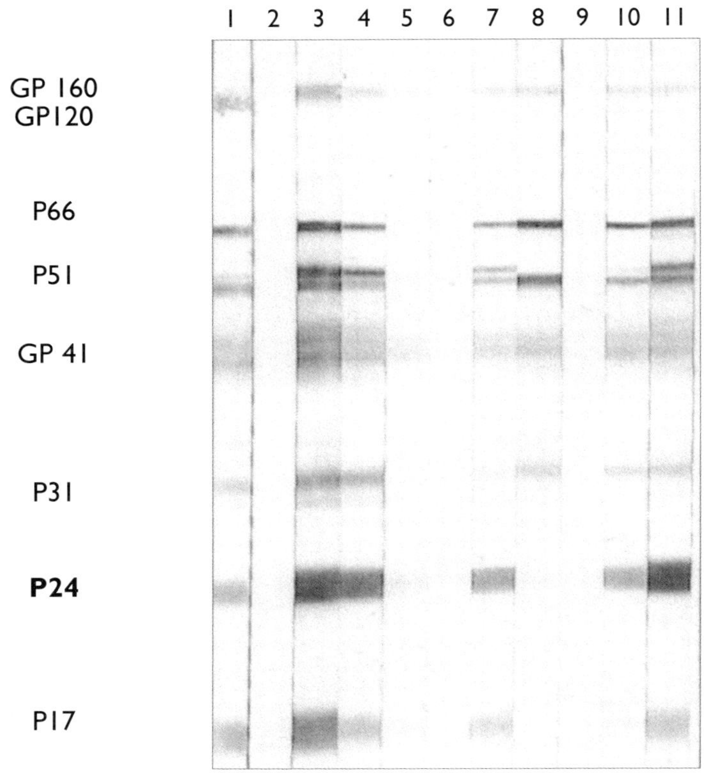

Fig. 9.3 The WB technique is designed to detect specific antibodies in the serum of patients that occur in autoimmune disease or in response to exogenous agents such as bacteria or viruses.

The various proteins of the suspected autoantigens or pathogen are isolated, denatured and separated by sodium dodecyl sulphate poly acrylamide gel electrophoresis (SDS-PAGE). SDS is a detergent that denatures proteins and imparts a negative charge to the denatured proteins and PAGE separates the proteins according to their molecular weights. The proteins in the gel are transferred to a nitrocellulose membrane which is then incubated with the patient's serum and any antibodies present will recognise and bind to it. After incubation and washing anti-human immunoglobulin linked with horse radish peroxidase and further washing the substrate is added and as with the ELISA technique the antibodies are shown up by a colour change. The bands are compared with bands derived from known positive and negative sera assayed on the same membranes. Lane one is a positive control and lane 2 a negative one - the others demonstrate antibodies in patients' sera.

The WB technique is of considerable value for the diagnosis of AIDS. The pattern of antibodies is characteristic of the disorder and represents the degree of immunological chaos that exists in this illness. With the knowledge that we now have that most preparations of the presumed external agent - HIV - consisted mostly of cellular material it seems clear that the AIDS WB test demonstrates above all that AIDS is an immunological disorder of the auto/alloimmune/GVH type. Studies on vaccines discussed later in this chapter indicate that a conventional external agent is not involved.

P24 is given prominence (bold) in the above depiction of the presumed antigens of HIV because it is also manifested in other autoimmune diseases such as SLE. In these other disorders that show anti-p24 activity there is a different pattern of antibodies overall and Deas *et al* (1998) have suggested that differing patterns of peptides could be syndrome specific and might prove to be useful diagnostic tools for SLE and related conditions.

Papadopulus-Eleopulos and her colleagues (2001) have written at length about the non-standardisation of these tests and have expressed considerable concern over the implications of misdiagnosis, especially in developing countries.

ANTI-P24 IN OTHER GVHD-LIKE IMMUNOPATHOLOGIES

Although no retroviruses *per se* have been found to be the cause of any of the classical human immuno-pathologies, antibodies to the AIDS p24 antigen have been. It is of considerable interest that these p24 antibodies have been demonstrated in those diseases that, like AIDS, possess a strong resemblance to GVHD.

In brief, Talal *et al* (1990, 1990a) found that 30% of SS and SLE patients reacted to p24 protein. Mason *et al* (1998) confirmed these results and also detected p24 sero-reactivity in 35% (27/77) of patients with primary biliary cirrhosis. A particularly interesting study by the Garry group (Deas *et al* 1998) on the occurrence of antibodies to the p24 antigen concerned both SLE and SS patients who had no evidence of exposure to AIDS. They examined and characterised the specific peptides involved in this cross-reactivity by means of an ELISA, and discovered characteristic epitope-specific profiles for SLE and SS patients and considered that the specificities could be syndrome specific and that further development of the assay techniques might result in useful diagnostic tools.

MOUSE MODELS

As in the case of the classic human GVHD-like immunopathologies, AIDS antibodies are found in GVHD/alloimmune mice (Kion and Hoffman (1991) (Fig 9.4). Allo-immune mice produced by injecting lymphocytes from each into the other in B6 and CBA strains of mice developed sero-positivity in what was effectively a positive AIDS test. Similar results were obtained in all eight hyper-immune allogenic mouse sera tested. The AIDS antigen gp 120 was demonstrated by the same authors in mice known as MRL/lpr/lpr, which are models for human SLE.

These observations support the idea that the AIDS p24 antigen is a widely conserved cellular one, which becomes apparent in GVHD, otherwise known as allo-immune disease (see microchimerism below). The occurrence of the characteristic 'AIDS' antibodies seems to be a result of the cell damage caused in the graft versus host (GVH) and host versus graft (HVG) conflict comparable in some respects to the mixed lymphocyte reaction (Chapter Six).

Fig. 9.4a The Occurrence of AIDS Antibodies p24 and gp120 in Allo-immune Mice Developed by Reciprocal Injection of Lymphocytes

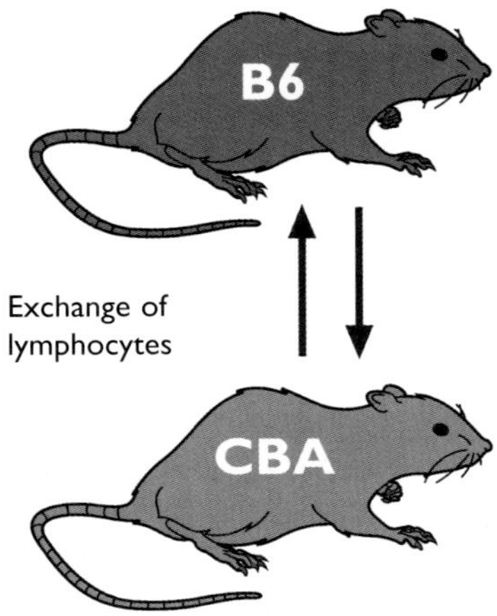

Alloimmune sera in pairs of strains of mice were raised by repeated reciprocal inoculations of lymphoid cells. The resulting sera tested by ELISA were found to contain antibodies to AIDS antigens p24 and gp 120. Similar results were obtained in all eight mouse allo-sera that were tested. The mice can be regarded as suffering from GVHD, which is similar to AIDS but which is caused by foreign /allo mouse cells - not by a virus.

Fig. 9.4b AIDS Antibodies in Mouse Models of Human SLE

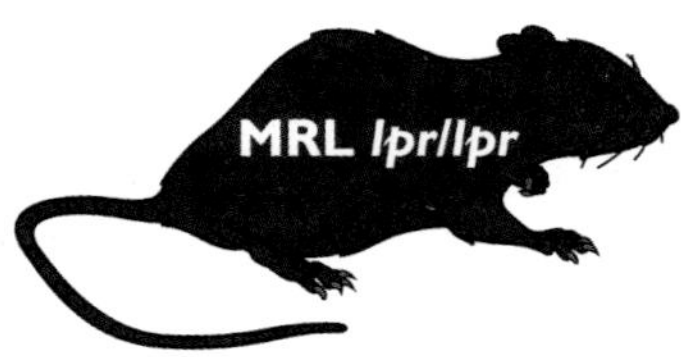

These MRL/lpr/lpr mice are models of the human disease SLE. They usually die at the age of six months from the progressive autoimmune disease and have many clinical and serological features in common not only with SLE patients but also those with AIDS. ELISA tests indicated that these mice also make anti-gp120 antibodies.

The development of this SLE mouse model began in 1976 (see Garry *et al* 1995) and involved the inbreeding of many strains of mice, a particular group of which after 12 generations developed massive lymph node enlargement early in life whilst others did not . Two sub-clones were developed, one with lymphadenopathy and severe Lupus, named MRL/l, and another that did not was named MRL/*n*. It was determined that the lymphadenopathy was controlled by a single recessive gene named the *lpr* gene.

MRL/*lpr* develop many of the signs and symptoms characteristic of human RA including swollen joints, development of rheumatoid factor, proliferation of synovial tissue and degradation of articular cartilage. Mice homozygous for *lpr* designated MRL/*lpr/lpr* are models for SLE and develop glomerulonephritis among other symptoms.

HUMAN TRANSPLANTATION AND P24

Organ transplantation in humans is effectively equivalent - although infinitely more tightly controlled - to the allo-grafting procedures carried out in animal laboratories, and if p24 is actually a cellular antigen incited by the presence of allo-material, it seems likely that the antigen would appear in some cases of organ transplantation in humans. There are at least two reports of transient p24 antigen occurring in the blood of recipients of organs from p24 antigen negative donors. (Papadopulos *et al* 2001).

SIMIAN AIDS AND VACCINES

The early work in this field, already mentioned in the previous chapter, was almost completely lacking in standard controls. The retrospective identification of an outbreak of a GVHD type of disease that had occurred in the Californian Primate research Centre as simian AIDS was hasty and ill-judged.

Normally an outbreak of an illness in an animal colony in which various procedures had been carried out on the animal population, manifesting itself as an immunodeficiency, in the form of opportunist infections and high-grade lymphomas, would be to look for GVHD as the probable cause. This would entail investigating the history of the animals to determine the possible source of the GVHD i.e. to determine whether the sick animals had been subjected to manipulations that had resulted in the engraftment of alien lymphocytes or related cells. This was not done (see below).

Kanki et al and Daniel et al (1985) working at the New England Regional Primate Centre (NERPC – see Fig. 9.6) claimed to have isolated a simian virus equivalent to HIV in humans that was cytopathogenic and contained proteins similar but not identical to those characteristic of HIV.

The techniques used for 'purification' of the virus-like particles were similar to those used for the 'purification' of HIV and it follows that the preparations of SIV were similarly compromised i.e. that the 'pure SIV' also consisted mostly of human cellular components, since the most of the work was carried out in the cell-lines H9 and HUT 78. Thus it comes as no surprise that SIV was found to be HIV related!

A further misinterpretation, was caused by the failure to control for mycoplasma contamination of the human cell-lines, which resulted in the attribution of cell-killing ability to the putative SIV instead of the mycoplasmas (Chapters 2 and 8)

Although the work on the macaque model is still regarded as constituting proof for the HIV equals AIDS concept, it is fair to say that the simian model itself was based on that assumption. In fact it is possible to argue that the reverse is the case and that the true worth of the work on SIV in macaques is that it virtually disproves the HIV=AIDS concept (see next page)

Fig. 9.5 A Macaque Monkey

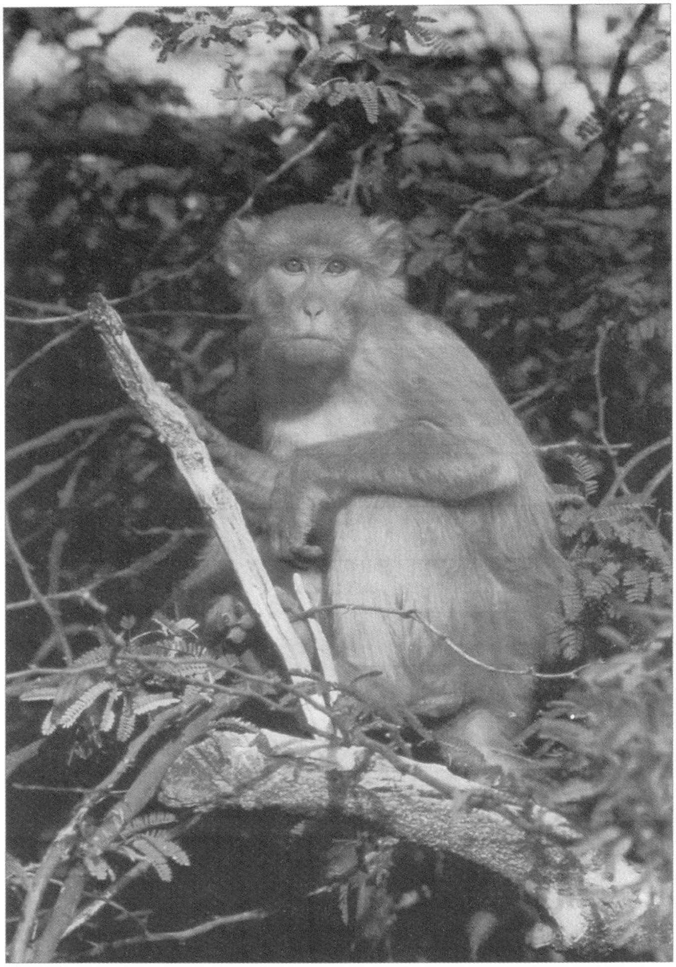

Fig. 9.5) This is a macaque monkey of the sort that was used in laboratories for investigations into diseases such as kuru and leprosy.

They were used for research into AIDS, particularly with a view to developing a prophylactic vaccine for humans, since they appeared to be suffering from a disease resembling human AIDS. However, on investigation of the origin of these animals it is apparent that some were survivors from GVH-like diseases that occurred in the late 60's and early 70's in a Primate Research Centre in California, which were sold on to different Centres where they were used for the AIDS research. Other macaques used in AIDS research, at the Delta Primate Centre at Tulane, were ones that had previously been inoculated with homogenates of a cutaneous leprosy lesion. Thus the macaques were immuno-compromised *before* they were used in AIDS research (Figs 9.6 and 9.7).

In fact, the use of macaques indicates very clearly that the 'simian immunodeficiency virus' (SIV) has nothing to do with the sickness suffered by the macaques, in spite of the presence of p24 sero-positivity, and the presence of virus-like particles. The work on vaccines, interpreted in a classic way, confirms this (Fig 9.6).

Reproduced from the Archives of the Royal Society for the Prevention of Cruelty to Animals UK, with permission.

LABORATORY HISTORY OF THE DAVIS MACAQUES

The illness that was later identified as simian 'AIDS' occurred at the Davis Primate Research Centre in California in 1969 and 1974. Apparently the macaques became ill shortly after they had been infected with kuru-infected human brain tissue, either directly, or with material from mangabey monkeys that had been used as intermediate hosts. This happened during research on 'slow viruses' by the Nobel laureate Carleton Gadjusek at the research centre in the fifties and seventies (Hooper 1999). Thus the surviving macaques were *already immunologically compromised* when sold on to other centres. The disorder persisted at some of these centres, and SIV was isolated from these affected animals (Fig 9.6). The macaque monkeys used for SIV isolation at the Delta Primate Centre at Tulane were also immunologically compromised (Fig. 9.7).

Fig. 9.6 History of the Macaque Monkeys Used in AIDS Research

Davis Primate Research Centre
California

Outbreaks of simian disease retrospectively identified as simian AIDS were observed in 1969 and 1974 during which time macaques had been inoculated with kuru-infected brain tissue, which had been passaged through mangabeys. The outbreak of simian-AIDS/GVHD followed.

→ Rhesus macaque survivors of the GVHD-like condition were dispatched to NERPRC in Boston New England and the condition perpetuated there and led to the identification of SIV after the similarities between AIDS and the macaque disease were recognised.

↓ Other survivors - long-tailed macaques *Macaca fascicularis* were sold on to the primate facility at Washington Seattle. Again the disease continued to appear and the work of Stott *et al* showing the efficacy of cellular vaccines was performed on *M. fascicularis*.

↓ In 1978 the colony of stump-tailed macaques was broken up and 4 were incorporated into a new stump-tail colony at YERKES situated near Atlanta.

Fig. 9. 7 Delta Primate Centre at Tulane

4 macaques developed AIDS-like illnesses after being inoculated with homogenates of a cutaneous lepromatous leprosy lesion from a sooty mangabey.

→ Injections of tissue homogenates from the 4 afflicted monkeys caused 'AIDS' in 11 out of 14 injected macaques. The AIDS antibody p24 was also present in these animals.

The authors (Murphey-Corb *et al* 1986) suggested that the macaque monkeys had been infected with the SIV/Delta virus (their 'isolate') from the mangabey monkeys, the difference in pathogenicity being due to the transfer of an African (mangabey) to an Asian (macaque) species. This explanation has stimulated studies concerning 'species jumps' from non-human primates to humans, but there is no proof that the jump from African to Asian monkeys caused the so-called simian AIDS.

The more likely explanation is that the occurrence of the sero-positivity to p24 and the 'AIDS' symptoms were due to the unfortunate macaques' response to alien mangabey cells. The virus-like particles identified as SIV are unrelated to the disease process (see below).

The second control failure in these experiments has already been touched upon in the last chapter, and concerns the failure to ensure that the viruses used for transmission experiments and for the preparation of vaccines were truly pure and not contaminated with cellular material arising from the tissue cultures in which the viruses were grown. It now seems clear that since the traditional unsound methods of retrovirus purification were used in these experiments, this factor needs to be taken into account in the interpretation of the experiments on these animals.

VACCINE STUDIES INDICATING THAT SIV DOES NOT CAUSE SIMIAN 'AIDS'

The classic work of Stott *et al* (1991), reported from Potters Bar UK, revealed the shortcomings of the early work on macaque monkeys and indicated that the real cause of the simian 'AIDS' was due to immunological conflict with human cellular material (later identified as HLA-II DR) and not the associated retrovirus SIV. Their investigations concerned the testing of SIV vaccines for their ability to protect macaques from simian AIDS, in the hope that a successful SIV vaccine could be the basis for a vaccine for the prevention in human AIDS.

In order to test the efficacy of the SIV vaccines, Stott *et al* 1991 followed the normal procedure by giving the macaques a course of injections of the virus, which had been inactivated so that it would not cause disease, but would still retain the ability to elicit protective antibodies in the recipient macaques. On completion of the course, the monkeys (four in each group) were then challenged with live virus (and as we now know, also with human cellular antigens).

The outstanding point about this research was that it included the use of control animals that were injected with uninfected cells of the same type that had been used to culture the SIV. The surprising result was that the vaccine made from uninfected cells protected the macaques from disease and death to the same extent as the protection afforded by the vaccine prepared from SIV infected cells. Further work showed that the higher the titre of antibodies to the cellular components, the greater was the protection afforded.

In brief, this work was of the utmost importance and had it been followed through seriously by the AIDS community, it might have brought about a change in the whole approach to the problem of the development of a vaccine for human AIDS, and avoided the *impasse* that exists today in that area.

The retrospective understanding that supposedly pure virus suspensions of retroviruses are contaminated with cellular materials enables a more accurate interpretation of these experiments to be made (Figs. 9.7 and 9.8).

Fig. 9.7 Diagrammatic Representation of Experiments on Macaques (After Stott et *al* 1991)

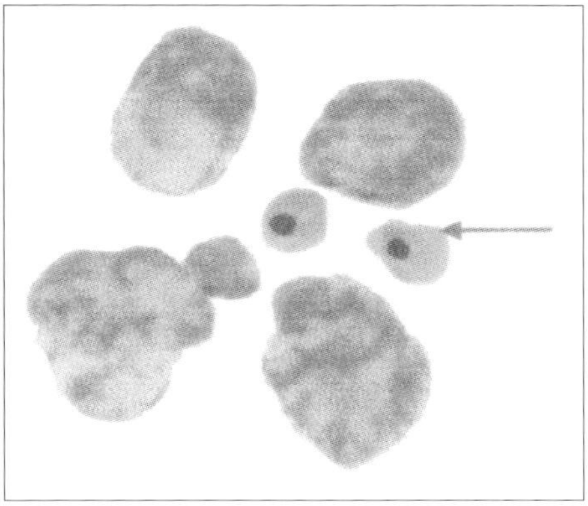

Vaccine prepared from what is now known to have been a mixture of virus particles identified as SIV (arrow) and human cellular components (Chapter Eight) was treated with gluteraldehyde and injected into macaques and it was found that the degree of protection that the vaccine provided was correlated with the antibody titres to the human cells ***i.e.*** the higher the titre to the human cellular antigens the greater was the protection. The antibodies to the supposed SIV can be explained by the fact that the cells in these preparations as opposed to the uninoculated ones below are damaged by GVHD reactions.

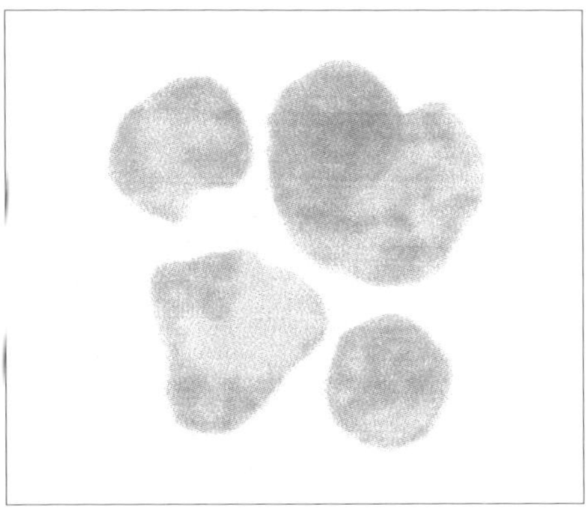

Vaccine prepared from uninoculated human cells alone protected the macaques from disease and death when challenged with live 'virus' preparations. This effectively exonerates the alleged causative agent - SIV - and indicates that the disorder in the macaques is laboratory-induced GVHD.

CONFIRMATION OF THE STOTT RESEARCH

The Bess *et al* 1997 paper, discussed in the previous chapter, emanated from the Frederick National Cancer Institute, Maryland, and was presumably stimulated by their previous important and elegant studies, which not only confirmed the observations of Stott *et al*, but also determined the nature of the cellular origin of the proteins that elicited the protective antibodies (Arthur *et al* 1995). These vital antibodies in the sera of the macaques that were protected from infection proved to be related to the HLA-II type of the cells in which the SIV was cultured.

The supreme importance of this protective role of antibodies to cellular HLA-II DR was very considerably highlighted by the group's observation that no such protection was afforded when the cells used for SIV growth were macaque PBMCs as opposed to the human H9 cells. Evidence of the disease process that occurred as a result of the injection of what was assumed to be purified SIV but which also must have contained macaque cellular material - possibly much in excess of SIV particles - was the detection of sero-positivity to gp 120. This indicates that some GVH reaction was occurring almost certainly as a result of the presence of the macaque class II antigens acting as allo-antigens *i.e.* class II antigens of the same species.

Arthur *et al* believed that the protection afforded to macaques by the Human Class II antibodies was total inasmuch as the antibodies presumed to be produced in response to infection by SIV were not present. In fact taking the view that simian 'AIDS' is a laboratory induced GVHD the protection afforded by the vaccine prepared from the human cell-line H9 is that it prevented the establishment of alien human clones in these vaccinated macaques. As I have already discussed such a GVHD situation results in the formation of antibodies to a mélange of autoantibodies produced in response to newly exposed antigens. This is what was prevented by the H9 vaccine and it is these auto-antibodies that have been misinterpreted as being responses to antigens that exist in SIV.

Fig. 9.8 Diagrammatic Representation and Interpretation of Experiments Showing that Simian 'AIDS' is a Laboratory-induced GVHD/alloimmunity, (After Arthur *et al* 1995)

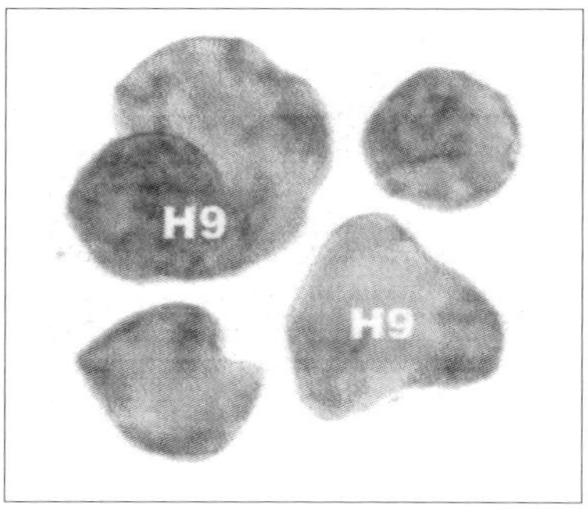

Control vaccine prepared from uninfected human cells (H9) processed as for virus isolation in sucrose gradients.

a)

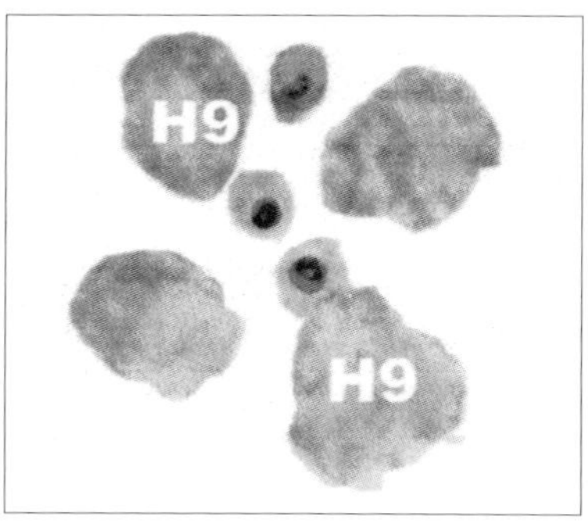

Macaques were given a course of injections of this vaccine after which they were challenged with

a) Live SIV grown in H9 (which will also include cellular components including HLA-II). If antibodies to the HLA-II have been produced in the macaque serum it is protected from infection.

b)

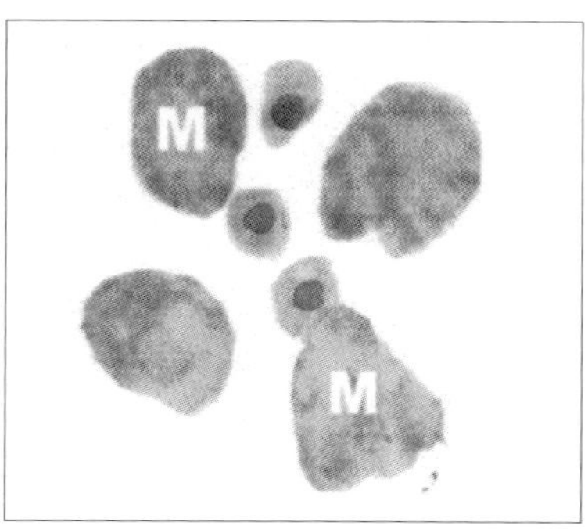

b) Live SIV grown in macaque PBMCs, which also contain simian class II antigens but no human ones. These animals are not protected and become infected. This shows that the protective factor was the formation of antibodies to the class II antigens contained in the tissue cells in which the virus- like particles were cultured.

As Arthur *et al* pointed out, this work indicates clearly that protection is solely due to the human class-II DR antigens (Fig. 9.8) and not to cross-reactive epitopes shared between MHC-encoded proteins and viral envelope glycoproteins.

Macaques were given immunisation courses with one of the following;

1) Control-vaccine prepared by harvesting the culture fluid from uninfected H9 cells and processing it by ultra-centrifugation in sucrose gradients in the same way that is used for HIV purification

2) Purified HLA-I I -DR protein prepared from H9. On challenge with intravenous infectious virus it was found that the macaques that had developed antibodies to H9 derived HLA-DR - in response to the purified HLA-II and the mock virus preparations - were protected from infection.

Vaccines prepared from H9 purified HLA-I elicited antibodies but did not afford protection from infection.

The macaques which were protected from challenge were given boosters of the same vaccines and challenged, this time with the same SIV but which was grown in macaque PBMCs as opposed to the human H9 cells. In this case all animals did become infected, indicating that the protection seen with human class II protein did not protect the macaques from infection with SIV containing macaque class II proteins.

GVHD - THE *MODUS OPERANDI* OF AIDS AND OTHER IMMUNOPATHOLOGIES

The work on simian AIDS and the classic electron-microscope studies on HIV/AIDS indicate that the extensive mimicry reputed to exist between HIV and cellular elements is an illusion, quite simply due to contamination. The presence of the cellular material in 'pure' HIV/SIV preparations is more than adequate to account for the cross-reactivity between auto-antibodies in a patient's/macaque's serum in AIDS/simian AIDS tests.

Further work from the Maryland laboratory (Esser *et al* 2000) makes no claim to have separated virus from cellular components; their findings can again be interpreted as demonstrating GVHD, with virus-like particles playing a small strictly mechanical part in the process. Esser *et al* mentioned that the mechanism responsible for the fact that HIV infection results in the non-functioning of CD4 cells happening a long time before their decline remains unclear. This is explicable in terms of the sero-conversion to p24 antibody positivity (a positive AIDS test) being the first indication of lymphocyte damage occurring at the beginning of GVHD, resulting in the emergence of endogenous p24 antigen. The possible contribution to this process by episomal DNA is discussed below.

Following this, the decline in numbers of CD4 cells is explicable in terms of the conflict mainly between the HLA-II antigens on the lymphocytes of endogenous origin and the differing HLA-II ones on the allo-lymphocytes that have found themselves in the afflicted animal through un-natural procedures such as therapeutic transplantation, transfusion of blood products, procedures involving the use of hypodermic syringes such as vaccination, and drug injection.

The risk of GVHD developing after blood transfusions in immunodeficient individuals has been known for over thirty years, but it is now recognised that in immuno-competent patients it is increased if the blood donor is genetically related and has closely related HLA components. This closeness or otherwise of HLA components appears to be of considerable importance in the natural chimerism (microchimerism) that occurs by the foetal maternal route.

MICROCHIMERISM, GVHD AND ALLO-IMMUNITY

The phenomenon of cell-trafficking that occurs in both directions between mother and foetus during pregnancy (Lo *et al* 1996) is a relatively new area of study and is known as microchimerism. The chimeric state in these conditions has come about through the natural occurrence of pregnancy, and various studies have shown links between the major factors under discussion; GVHD/chimerism; Auto/allo immune disease and the importance of HLA types in these phenomena.

Foetal cells in maternal blood were first clearly demonstrated by Herzenberg *et al* in 1979 and seventeen years later in the course of investigating methods of non-invasive techniques for the detection of foetal chromosome abnormalities. Bianchi *et al* (1996) made the surprising discovery that foetal cells representative of haemopoietic progenitors of the type with the potential to develop into a lymphoid cell-line (Chapters Six and Seven) can exist in women for as long as twenty-seven years after pregnancy.

This observation led to the idea that microchimerism might provide a clue as to why the GVHD-like diseases such as SLE SS and especially scleroderma (Nelson 1996) are much more prevalent in women than in men. In this paper, Nelson adduced evidence for the probable involvement of HLA relationships being of importance in microchimerism. This was partly based on the observation (Nelson *et al* 1993) that the well-known improvement that is often experienced by women with arthritis during pregnancy is related to the degree of compatibility with that of the developing foetus. Disparity between mother and foetus was associated positively with improvement in the arthritic symptoms.

There have been several studies on the possible role of microchimerism in scleroderma (SSc) and generally speaking the overall impression is that patients show a higher degree of the microchimerism than control subjects, and there is a tendency for there to be a correlation between the occurrence of the disease and HLA compatibility with the foetus, reminiscent of the blood-transfusion GVHD cases mentioned above.

Nelson *et al* 1998 investigated the occurrence of male-chromosome-specific sequences in the peripheral blood of women with SSc and in healthy ones, who had given birth to a son or sons, to determine the number of male DNA equivalents in each group, and found that the numbers were significantly higher in the SSc patients. Moreover, they found that Class II HLA compatibility was more common for SSc patients than for controls. Women with SSc were found to be nine times more likely to have given birth to a child compatible for HLA DRB-I genes, and the risk is increased nineteen-fold if the child is compatible. Several reviews are available on this subject, including Lambert *et al* (2001) and Igaz (2000).

Clearly microchimerism cannot be the only factor in autoimmune disease in women, since it also occurs in healthy ones. However, HLA compatibility is clearly an important factor, and it is possible that maternal-foetal transfer of the human endoparasite, and/or other microorganisms, is involved (Chapters Three and Seven).

THE TRANSMISSION OF AIDS

From the beginning of the AIDS epidemic it has been realised that its marked GVHD aspects were difficult to explain without some clear means of the transfer and engraftment of the putative invading alien cells. The possibility that the more invasive gay practices combined with drug-induced immunosuppression exists in theory but this clearly does not apply in most cases.

The problem of the transmissibility of the disorder seemed to have been solved by the discovery of HIV but as I have tried to point out, this scenario is not really credible and it seems that although many serious establishment AIDS investigators are not entirely happy with the simple HIV=AIDS concept the lack of a plausible alternative has led to the maintenance of the *status quo*.

In spite of the urging of Fields (Chapter Eight) to search for new paradigms and conceptual frameworks, especially those of other microbial life-styles that could provide insight into the AIDS problem, no attempts have so far been made. I have already proposed an NGE for AS, which might be described as an HLA Class I immunopathology and here I am suggesting a similar framework for the ones in which the HLA- class II DR antigens are involved. The diseases in question, which can conveniently be described as belonging to the collagen group - e.g. AIDS, SLE, SS, and RA and the first three of these have strong affinities with GVHD.

Since the damage caused in the classic collagen disorders can be organ or tissue specific, or can occur on a wider scale with varying degrees of systemic involvement, it is also necessary to postulate coding for tropism sequences. The variations in the composition of the putative episomes could account for the variations in the course and severity of the disorders, which may have a rapid and life-threatening course or a chronic, slowly progressive, relatively benign one. Although theoretically an infinite variety of episome sequence variations is possible, some combinations would prove more viable than others, so that a statistically significant number of cases of infection would show groups of clinical features that represent the better-known syndrome.

P24 AND THE PROPOSED AIDS EPISOME COMPOSITION

I have discussed at length in the last chapter the possibility that the AIDS antigen p24 is a widely conserved cellular antigen and that the p24 AIDS antibody test is a test for an autoantibody and not a response to an outside agent.

In fact, the episome theory allows for the possibility that it could be both, in the same way that the HLA-II endogenous and exogenous (as part of the putative episome DNA) does (Fig. 9.9).

Fig. 9.9 Suggested *Modus Operandi* of Episome Infection in AIDS

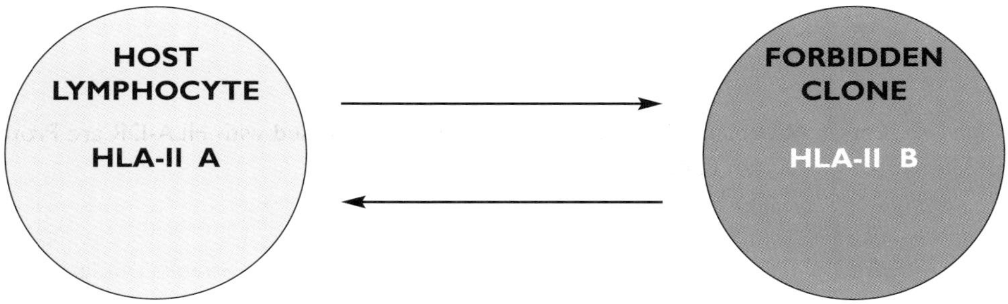

The infecting episome DNA in this case contains some coding for HLA II DR and for CD 4 tropism. Cells are probably infected early in the process of haemopoiesis and then multiply, forming, in the terminology of Burnet, a 'forbidden clone', which recognises the host cells as foreign and reacts against them in the classic GVH manner. The host cells also react against the forbidden clone cells and the conflict begins. During this time the classic p24 antibody becomes exposed gradually, depending on the intensity of the conflict - this is influenced by the degree of difference that exists between the HLA II antigens involved. This would explain the discrepancy between the time of appearance of the p24 sero-positivity and the onset of the decline in CD 4 cells.

The electron-micrograph of MNCL 4 (Bess *et al* Chapter Eight) provides a good basis for discussion of this point. Clone 4 was derived from a single cell, originally from the H9 cell-line, which was rich in p24, and the possibility exists that this was a damaged cell still capable of reproduction (perhaps particularly able as is the case with malignant cells). It is interesting in this context that the p24 production was lower in the sub-cultures of these into cell-lines of different origins, which is likely to cause more destruction due to differing HLA specificities. This explanation is in accordance with the view that p24 is only a product of GVHD, However, the preparation shows a fairly impressive number of virus-like particles, and this suggests that these could be an alternative source of p24 and this suggests that some form of p24 constitutes part of the theoretical AIDS episome.

SUMMARY

It is pointed out that the immunopathologies under discussion *i.e.* the classic 'autoimmunities', and AIDS have certain features in common, some of which provide clues to the underlying aetiologies. These include HLA-disease connections, GVHD and molecular mimicry. In the case of AIDS particularly but not exclusively, the 'AIDS' protein p24 is of obvious importance, at least in diagnosis, and this as well as 'AIDS' tests and their significance is also discussed.

The problems with the macaque monkey models for human AIDS, with special reference to the work suggesting that the proposed aetiological agent - SIV - is not involved in simian AIDS and the question of what bearing this has on the HIV/AIDS concept are addressed.

The concept of allo/immunity mediated by foreign DNA (episome/plasmid) that I have previously proposed for the classic immunopathologies is revised and a similar mechanism for the aetiology of AIDS is tentatively proposed.

REFERENCES

Arthur, L.O., Bess, J.W. Urban, R.G. *et al* (1995) Macaques Immunised with HLA-DR are Protected from Challenge with Simian Immunodeficiency Virus
Journal of Virology 69 3117-3124

Bess, J.W., Gorelick, R.J. Bosche, W.J. *et al* (1997) Microvesicles are a Source of Contaminating Cellular Proteins found in Purified HIV-1 Preparations
Virology 230 134-144

Bianchi, D.W., Zickwolf, G.K., Weil, G.J. *et al* (1996) Male fetal progenitor cells persist in maternal blood for as long as 27 years post-partum
Proc.Natl.Acad. Sci. U.S. 93 705-708

Bianchi, D.W. (2000) Feto-maternal Cell Trafficking: A New Cause of Disease?
American Journal of Medical Genetics 91 22-28

Burnet, M. (1962) The Integrity of the Body
Harvard University Press London: Oxford University Press

Cameron, F.H., Russell, P.J., Sullivan, J. *et al* (1983) Is a Klebsiella plasmid involved in the aetiology of ankylosing spondylitis in HLA-B17 positive individuals?
Mol Immunl 20 563-566

Daniel M.D., Letvin N.L., King N. W. *et al* (1985) Isolation of a T-Cell Tropic HTLV-111-Like Retrovirus from Macaques *Science* 228 1201-1204

Dalgleish, A.G. (1992) The pathogenesis of AIDS: classical and alternative views
Journal of the Royal College of Physicians of London 26 152-158

Deas, J.E., Liu, L.G., Thompson, J.J. *et al* (1998) Reactivity of Sera from Systemic Lupus Erythematosus and Sjogren's Syndrome Patients with Peptides Derived from Human Immunodeficiency Virus p24 Capsid Antigen
Clinical and Diagnostic Laboratory Immunology 5 181-185

Ebringer, A., Wilson, C. and Tiwana, H. (2000) Is Rheumatoid Arthritis a Form of Reactive Arthritis?
The Journal of Rheumatology 27 560-563 editorial.

Edmonds, J. Geczy, A.F. Sullivan, J.S. *et al* (1983) Enteric Bacteria and HLA-B27 Associated Cell Surface Modification in Patients with Sero-negative Spondarthritis
Brit.J. Rheumatol. 22 (Suppl 2) 75-84

Garry, R.F., Kreig, A.M., Cheevers, W.P. (1995) Retroviruses and Their Roles in Chronic Inflammatory Diseases and Autoimmunity
The Retroviridae, 4 491-602

Geczy, A. F., Alexander., K. and Bashir, H. V. *et al* (1980) A factor(s) in *Klebsiella* culture filtrates specifically modifies an HLA-B27-associated surface component
Nature 283 782-784

Ginsberg, H.S. (1980) Togaviruses, Bunyaviruses and Arenaviruses In Microbiology 3rd Ed. Edits Davis B.D., Dulbecco, R., Eisen, H.N. Ginsberg, H.S.

Gougeon, M-L., and Montagnier L. (1993) Apoptosis in AIDS
Science 260 1269-1270

Gougeon, M-L, Garcia, S. Heeney J., *et al* (1993) Programmed cell death in AIDS-related and SIV infections
AIDS Res Hum Retroviruses Jun; 9 (6) 553-563

Habeshaw, J.A. and Dalgleish, A.G. (1989) The Relevance of HIV env/CD4 Interactions to the Pathogenesis of Acquired Immune Deficiency Syndrome
Journal of Acquired Immune Deficiency Syndromes 2 457-468

Herzenberg, L. A., Bianchi, D. W., Schroder, J. *et al* (1979) Foetal cells in the blood of pregnant women: detection and enrichment by fluorescence-activated cell sorting
Proc Natl Acad Sci USA 76 1453-1455

Hooper, E. (1999) The River
Allen Lane The Penguin Press

Igaz,P. (2000) Foetal cells and the pathogenesis of scleroderma - microchimerism and mechanisms of allo-immunity
Wien Med Wochenschr 150 101-2 (in German)

Kanki P. J., McLane M.F., King N.W. *et al* (1985) Serologic Identification and Characterisation of a Macaque T-Lymphotropic Retrovirus Closely Related to HTLV-111
Science 228 1199-1201

Kion T.A and Hoffmann G.W. (1991) Anti-HIV and Anti-Anti-MHC Antibodies in Alloimmune and Autoimmune Mice
Science 253 1138

Lambert, N.C., Stevens, A.M., Tylee, T.S. *et al* (2001) From the Simple Detection of Microchimerism in Patients with Autoimmune Diseases to its Implication in Pathogenesis
Ann. N.Y. Acad Sci. 945 164-171

Lo. D.Y.M., Watson, N., Noakes, L. *et al* (1996) Two-way traffic between mother and foetus : biological and clinical implications
Blood 88 4390-4395

MacKintosh, P. and Pease, P. (1982) HLA-B27, Ankylosing Spondylitis and some normal Rabbit Sera
Ann. Rheum. Dis. 41 433-434

Maddox J. AIDS research turned upside down (1991)
Nature 353 297

Mason, A.L., Xu, L. Guo, L *et al* (1998) Detection of retroviral antibodies in primary biliary cirrhosis and other idiopathic biliary disorders
Lancet 351 1620-1624

Montagnier, L. (2000) 'virus'
W.W. Norton & Company New York London

Murphey-Corb M., Martin L.M., Rangan S.R.S *et al* (1986) Isolation of an HTLV-111-related retrovirus from macaques with simian AIDS and its possible origin in asymptomatic mangabeys
Nature 321 435-437

Nelson, J.L., Fuerst, D.E., Maloney, S. *et al* (1998) Microchimerism and HLA compatible relationships of pregnancy in scleroderma
Lancet 351 559-562

Nelson. J.L., Hughes, K. A. Smith, A.G. *et al* (1993) Maternal-foetal disparity in HLA class 11 allo-antigens and the pregnancy-induced amelioration of rheumatoid arthritis
N Eng J Med 329 466-471

Nelson, J. (1996) Maternal-Foetal Immunology and Autoimmune Disease: Is some Autoimmune Disease Auto-Alloimmune or Allo-Autoimmune?
Arthritis and Rheumatism 39 191-194

Papadopulos-Eleopulos, E., Turner, V. F. Papadimitriou, J. M. *et al* (2001) Mother to Child Transmission of HIV and its Prevention with AZT and Nevirapine: A critical Analysis of the Evidence
North American Edition: Alberta Reappraising AIDS Society.

Pease, P E. (1965) L-Forms, Episomes and Autoimmune Disease
E. & S, Livingstone Ltd, Edinburgh and London

Pease, P.E., England, J., Tyler, R. *et al* (1980) HLA-B27, Yersinia enterocolitica and ankylosing spondylitis
Ann.Rheum Dis 39 415-416

Pease, P.E. (1984) A reappraisal of the episome theory of autoimmune disease in the light of evidence from various sources
Rivista di Biologia 77 13-33

Pease, P.E., Balmer, S.E., Tallack, J.E. *et al* (1986) Further observations upon HLA-B27, Yersinia enterocolitica and ankylosing spondylitis
Ann. Rheum. Dis. 45 526-528
Shearer, G.(1983) A clinician and a scientist look at AIDS – A consequence of allogenic la-antigen recognition
Immunology Today 4 181-182

Stastny, P. (1978) Association of the B-cell alloantigen DrW4 with rheumatoid arthritis
N Eng J Med 287 869-871

Stott, E.J. (1991) Anti-cell antibody in macaques
Nature 353 393

Tiwana, H., Wilson, C. Walmsley, R. S. *et al* (1997) Antibody responses to gut bacteria in ankylosing spondylitis, rheumatoid arthritis, Crohn's Disease and ulcerative colitis
Rheum Int 17 11-16

Thomas, L. (1992) As quoted by Duesberg - AIDS acquired by Drug Consumption and other Non-Contagious Risk Factors
Pharmac. Ther 55 201-277

Wilson, C., Tiwana, H. and Ebringer, A. (2000) Molecular mimicry between HLA-DR alleles associated with rheumatoid arthritis and Proteus mirabilis as the aetiological basis for autoimmunity
Microbes and infection 2 1489-1496

AFTERWORD

‘I do not know any country where, in general, less independence of mind and genuine freedom of discussion reign than in America.

'Only foreigners or experience can make certain truths reach the ears of the American.'

'In America the majority draws a formidable circle around thought. Inside those limits the writer is free; but unhappiness awaits him if he dares to leave them.'

De Tocqueville (1831)

‘The anonymous New York Times wordsmith was not an innocent abroad. He knew exactly what he was doing. He was trying to nobble the jury, complementing the word ‘spin’ (as in ‘to spin a yarn’ or perhaps as in spin bowling in cricket), with the word ‘doctor’ (meaning to titivate, tamper with and even falsify) in order to brand with the mark of Cain all those in the business of liaising with and guiding journalists.’

Bernard Ingham, press officer to Margaret Thatcher (2003)

There have been hundreds of thousands of publications on AIDS and HIV - the connection is so well-established that the terms have become interchangeable and yet very strong evidence exists that the connection is a mistake. Furthermore it seems to me that this can be demonstrated by a serious look at twelve key papers.

KEY PAPERS

Bold provide valuable information - Regular provide misleading material.

1) Montagnier group (1983). The merit of this paper lies in the important discovery of the 'AIDS antigen' p24 which elicits antibodies in the serum of AIDS patients and those at risk of AIDS. Persons with this antibody are called sero-positive. The group tentatively suggested that the virus-like particles they observed might be the cause of AIDS. Since the publication of this work Montagnier has repeatedly said that HIV is not enough to cause AIDS. (Chapters Two and Eight)

2) Gallo *et al* (1984). Actually this work was separated into four papers, which appeared a year later and followed up the Paris ones. They are of very poor quality - the experiments were uncontrolled and unfortunately misled vast numbers of other investigators. The impression given was that they provided proof of the causative relationship between HIV and AIDS, and work claiming to verify this assumption (such as Darby *et al,* see below) has been based on the assumption that what they are attempting to prove is in fact true.

3) Darby *et al* (1995). This paper was greeted with enthusiasm, particularly by the press, and indeed at first sight it appeared impressive. However, closer examination reveals that it is based on the assumption that p24 sero-positivity means HIV infection, as assumed, but not proven to be true, by Gallo *et al*. Furthermore, no attempt was made to ascertain the role of haemoplasmas and related bacteria. (Chapter Three)

4) Montagnier group (1990). This is a real classic - demonstrating that the cell-killing properties of the supposed HIV were in fact due to contaminating mycoplasmas. (Chapters Two and Eight)

5) and 6) Ho *et al* and Wei *et al* (1995). These workers attempted to explain the fact that HIV is not cytopathogenic *per se* by suggesting that it is so pathogenic that cell annihilation of CD-4 cells is so rapid and cell replacement so efficient that it is not possible to detect the destruction in the normal way. This explanation is no longer valid. (Wolthers *et al* - see below). The urging of rapid retroviral treatment at sero-conversion to p24 positivity is fortunately no longer advised. (Chapter Eight)

7) Wolthers et al (1998). This group produced evidence, which demonstrated that CD-4 turnover in AIDS is not especially high, and that the Ho and Wei papers mentioned above give a false picture of AIDS.(Chapter Eight)

8) Kion and Hoffman (1991). These workers demonstrated that 'AIDS' antibodies p24 and gp 120 occur in allo-immune mice with no virus involved, providing a strong clue to the endogenous nature of the eliciting antigenic components.(Chapter Eight)

9) Stott et al (1991). This is another true classic that has not received the attention it deserved - it is short but absolutely critical. It reported that vaccines prepared from cellular material only, i.e. without the putative infective agent, protected macaques from so-called simian AIDS. It was a considerable improvement upon previous work carried out by other workers inasmuch as control macaques were used in these experiments. However Stott et al relied on the techniques developed by previous investigators for the 'isolation' of retroviruses and were unaware that their 'purified SIV' consisted mainly of cellular materials.(Chapter Nine)

10) Arthur et al (1995). This group provided evidence for the non-involvement of SIV in the macaque illness. They found that macaques vaccinated with human cells were protected from challenge with SIV (actually human cells plus a few virus-like particles - see below). The essential protective element was human lymphocyte antigen (HLA-DR) and this was the main point made in the paper. However the more significant observation, hardly mentioned by the authors, was that macaques challenged by SIV grown in macaque cells (PBMCs) (actually consisting of macaque cells and a few virus-like particles) were not protected. This demonstrates unequivocally that the protection is against allo/antigens and nothing to do with the virus-like particles aka SIV. (Chapter Nine)

It seems that the true value of the macaque model of human AIDS has been to show that the HIV=AIDS concept is wrong and to highlight the hopelessness of the search for a vaccine based on it.

11) and 12.) Bess et al and Gluschankof et al. (1997). These are the two classic papers that prove that HIV has never been separated from cellular components and reinforce the work on SIV and macaques to the point of proof that HIV is not responsible for AIDS. (Chapter Eight)

The implications of this with respect to therapy and prevention are of course incalculable and need to be assessed very seriously. First however, it is necessary to return to the beginning of the AIDS epidemic in order to gain some insight into how this situation arose.

1984 HIV, SPIN DOCTORING AND THE ORWELLIAN NIGHTMARE

1984 was the year of the birth of spin-doctoring (Ingham 2003), of Orwell's predicted commencement of the totalitarian nightmare, and also the year of the promotion of the idea of the American discovery of HIV as the cause of AIDS, with the promise of a vaccine for its prevention within two years. It is now clear that both these latter pronouncements were mistakes.

Nevertheless the concept of HIV continues and the epidemic is said to be progressing relentlessly and is now out of control.

From the beginning of the AIDS campaign, intelligence warnings were ignored or rejected - a fatal thing in war, as the fight against AIDS might be described (Regan 1987). This rejection of unpalatable intelligence concerning the problems with the HIV=AIDS concept, notably supplied by a highly respected retrovirologist until then - Peter Duesberg - can be constructively compared with the Japanese attack on Pearl Harbour in December 1941. Warnings had been issued weeks and months before concerning this, but these were not heeded and analysed, and the cost of this was incalculable. The current world-wide problem of AIDS has some alarming parallels.

Further very serious doubts cast on the role of HIV (above) have also remained unanswered by the AIDS establishment, and it is difficult to disagree with the conclusion that outside the formidable circle (de Tocqueville 1831), of the AIDS establishment in this case, persons putting forward different views in the US are *persona non grata*. Thus Duesberg has been the target of spin and been cast as dangerous, and he has been totally side-lined. Non-American dissenters have been ignored. President Mbeki of South Africa has been cast as a villain. It seems that the American 'formidable circle' has indeed succeeded in eliminating all dissent with respect to the HIV=AIDS concept even when the dissent is well-informed.

The almost universal acceptance of the belief that HIV is the sole cause of AIDS is arguably a feat of marketing - an area in which America has truly led the world. Such market forces would be kept in check if a healthy democracy were in place, but it now seems that 'Big Money' rules in America. Big money, it seems, calls the tune - it allows ownership of the media, and this for the most part ensures control of information made available to the public. Big money can also control the scientists it employs and the content of their publications.(see also Rasnick 2001 and Jacques 2004).

Thus the HIV concept has been sold as established truth in spite of evidence to the contrary, so effectively that there is now a world-wide demand for 'anti-retroviral' drugs and for a prophylactic vaccine.

Paradoxically, the fact is that AIDS, which began as a small allegedly controllable epidemic, has now become a pandemic for which no truly long-term effective therapy has been found and no effective vaccine has emerged. This has led, not to a reconsideration of the role of HIV in AIDS, but to an increase in funding and investment for the search for almost certainly unattainable goals.

The good side of the marketing expertise is the promotion of condom use. It needs to be reiterated here that NO RESPONSIBLE MICROBIOLOGIST WOULD ADVOCATE UNPROTECTED, PROMISCUOUS SEX UNDER ANY CIRCUMSTANCES.

However, where AIDS is concerned, condom use may not be the whole answer. For example, it appears that in places such as Zimbabwe, where condom use has brought about a 25% reduction in sexually-transmitted diseases (STDs) in high-risk groups, prostitutes, young people, lorry drivers *etc* - there has been a 12% increase in p24 sero-positivity (Brewer, D. *et al* (2003), Gisselquist, D., Potterat, *et al* (2003).

Recent work carried out by these research workers (from several universities) has provided impressive evidence, indicating that the heterosexual route has been grossly exaggerated and that iatrogenic factors have been very much underestimated.

WOMEN, AIDS AND HETEROSEXUAL TRANSMISSION

The work of Gisselquist and his colleagues constitutes the first serious reappraisal in 25 years of the received wisdom that AIDS in Africa is primarily a heterosexually transmitted disease, the main risk factor being 'the degree of sexual activity with multiple partners'. This view stems from the work of Piot (now the Executive Director of the United Nations AIDS campaign - UNAIDS) - (Piot *et al* 1988).

This implies that Africans practice the life-styles characteristic of gays in the early stages of the epidemic, and it seems that this interpretation of Piot's results may have been influenced by the wish to remove the impression that AIDS is a gay disease. In the words of Gisselquist *et al* 2003 discussed below, Piot's interpretation may have had 'more to do with political savvy than science'.

Whatever the pressures of political correctness influencing the Piot *et al* work implying that AIDS is not a gay disease, the situation now according to him, speaking on the part of UNAIDS 2004, is that women are now firmly at the centre of the epidemic. It is estimated that a higher percentage of women are sero-positive than men - some estimates put the percentage of sero-positive women as over 60 percent. UNAIDS have claimed that these figures have made the issue a women's rights one and this is most certainly the case.

UNAIDS has also claimed that women are biologically more likely to be infected than men and this clearly needs further clarification, since anal intercourse is much more dangerous for disease transmission than is vaginal, a fact that can be accounted for by the robustness of the vaginal as opposed to the anal lining.

This view is consistent with the findings of the Gisselquist group who cited evidence indicating that the rates of heterosexual transmission of p24/AIDS are 'remarkably similar' in the West and in Africa, except where compounding factors, such as unorthodox sexual practices, are present. It will be recalled, also, (Chapter Eight) that Peterman *et al* found only a small percentage of cases of the transfer of p24 sero-positivity between spouses. Clearly, other factors must be taken into account in assessing the nature of the biological role of women referred to by UNAIDS.

It seems certain that the main reason for female vulnerability lies in their role as mothers and that when pregnant they are subjected to all kinds of potentially dangerous medical interventions (see below) carried out in the name of protection of their babies. Since the offspring will consist of males as well as females, it means that much of the future of Africans of both sexes will be endangered.

Paradoxically, support for the role of the iatrogenisis concept of AIDS comes from studies on African women of high social status and education. These factors correlate with increased cases of p24/AIDS in women in parts of Africa and this would explain the higher incidence of p24/AIDS in women who have been seen in prenatal, *post partum* and induced abortion settings than in their community counterparts (Downs, *et al* 1996; Brewer *et al* 2004).

DANGER OF 'AIDS' DRUGS TO WOMEN AND THEIR BABIES

The first drug used for the treatment of patients was AZT, which is highly toxic (Fig. A1) and which was administered to healthy p-24 positive gay males in the early days of the AIDS epidemic. There is some considerable concern about this practice, expressed most notably by Duesberg, that it actually causes the symptoms that characterise AIDS. The implication here is that AIDS is a drug-induced disease.

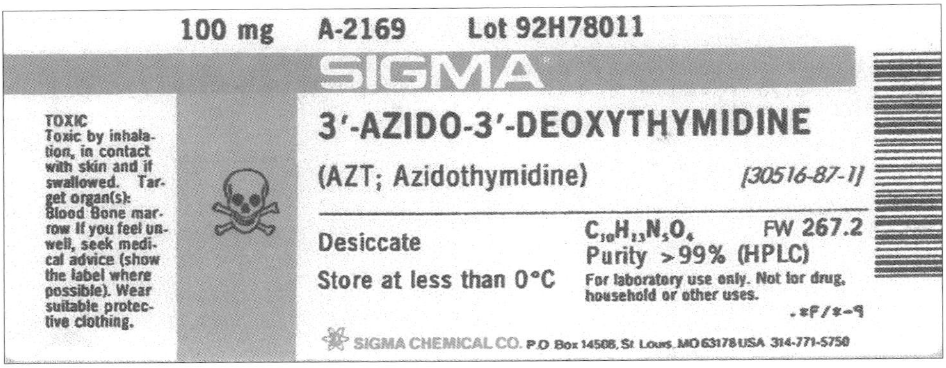

Fig. AI - The perceived urgency of the AIDS epidemic led to a hasty attempt to find a treatment for the condition, and AZT (3'-azide-3-deoxythymidine *aka* zidovudine and retrovir), which was initially developed for the treatment of the putative retrovirus cause of cancer (Chapter Five), led to a reconsideration of its use against the 'new retrovirus' believed to cause AIDS.

After endorsement by the FDA, Burroughs Wellcome applied for and obtained a patent for it, and it was administered to symptom-less p24 positive individuals in spite of its extreme toxicity.

Duesberg (1995) considers that the trials leading to the FDA endorsement were unsatisfactory and that the advanced AIDS that developed was due to the drug and not to the virus.

Notwithstanding the toxicity of the drug, it is used to treat pregnant African women and their babies in the belief that it will prevent the transmission of AIDS to babies.

I have pointed out (Chapter Nine) that the occurrence of p24 sero-positivity in gays could be a self-limiting GVH effect and, if this is the case, then it seems almost certain that the AZT was responsible for many of the AIDS deaths in the early days of the epidemic. The introduction of the less toxic HAART therapy has for the most part replaced AZT and comparable drugs in the West, but not so far in countries of the developing world to any extent.

This aspect of women, babies and AIDS is the subject of a comprehensive monograph - 'Mother to Child Transmission of HIV and its Prevention with AZT and Nevirapine' written by the Perth Group. This careful and thorough analysis of the evidence clearly shows that the administration of these drugs to pregnant women and their offspring is not only completely ineffective but actually dangerous to both mother and child. Their criticisms are based mainly on the lack of controls and generally poor design of the trials e.g. in some cases placebos were lacking and sometimes toxic placebos were used and when treatment did not produce expected results this was put down, as usual, to mutation of the putative virus. The group also emphasized the differences in protocols for testing experimental designs (Fig. A2) and was highly critical of the methods used for the determination of the alleged HIV infection. This suggests that there is a strong possibility that testing for the supposed AIDS antigen is often unsound (Chapter Nine).

Fig. A.2 Criteria used to define a positive HIV western blot

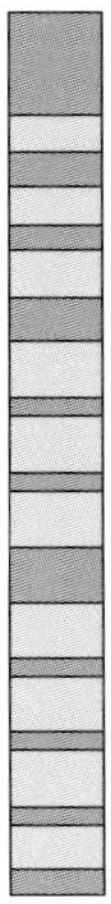

HIV WESTERN BLOT STRIP*	AFR	AUS	FDA	RCX	CDC 1	CDC 2	CON	GER	UK	FRA	MAC
ENV: p160, p120, p41	ANY 2	ANY 1	ANY 1	ANY 1	p160/ p120 AND p41	p160/ p120 AND p41	p160/ p120 AND p41	ANY 1	ANY 1	ANY 3	3 WEAK BANDS OR ANY STRONG BAND
POL: p68, p53, p32; *GAG*: p55, p39, p24, p18		ANY 3 GAG OR POL	p32 AND p24	ANY 1 AND ANY 1		AND p24	p32 OR p24	ANY 1 GAG OR POL	p32 AND p24	ANY 1 AND ANY 1	

AFR=AFRICA; AUS=AUSTRALIA; FDA=US FOOD AND DRUG ADMINISTRATION; RCX=US RED CROSS; CDC=US CENTRE FOR DISEASE CONTROL; CON=US CONSORTIUM FOR RETROVIRUS SEROLOGY STANDARDIZATION; GER=GERMANY; UK=UNITED KINGDOM; FRA=FRANCE; MACS=US MULTICENTER AIDS COHORT STUDY 1983-1992 *Bands not in electrophoretic order.

The occurrence of p24 sero-positivity in children with sero-negative mothers, which could not be attributed to vertical transmission, can also be attributed to medical intervention.

NON-SEXUAL ROUTES OF TRANSMISSION IN AIDS

The other main risk group apart from the gay population in developed countries is intravenous drug users (IDUs).

Obviously, recreational drug use was not the cause of the African epidemic, but mass vaccination programs clearly provided a non-sexual route for possible transmission. In these programs, which were carried out before the onset of AIDS, injections were given to men, women and children.

The first suspicions that vaccination programs could be related to the onset of AIDS were voiced by Wright (1987) and concerned the anti-smallpox campaign. There was evidence that some 50,000 deaths from AIDS were concentrated in the countries where the smallpox immunisation program was most intensive. Moreover, the smallpox campaign ended in 1980 – just when the AIDS epidemic came to be recognised. This important possibility was rejected by the WHO on the grounds of shortage of evidence. There has been no effort to search for more, so this factor cannot truly be excluded from the AIDS scenario.

Later, some anecdotal evidence along these lines was provided by Hooper (1999) who wrote 'I had reliable reports about un-sterilised needles being jabbed into arm after arm during the smallpox campaigns in the early 60s'. In fact, Hooper believed that the earlier anti-polio campaign was responsible for the AIDS epidemic, but the principle is the same – that the third, hitherto unacknowledged factor in the AIDS epidemic is the hypodermic syringe, which provides a mechanism which, whatever the exact cause, can allow the cause of AIDS to pass from one person to another other than by the sexual route..

Whatever the truth of the role of the smallpox eradication program in AIDS, it does seem likely that supposed heath-care measures when carried out by poorly trained individuals can actually cause ill-health.

This could very well account for the anecdotal stories of whole villages being wiped out by AIDS in China. The simplest answer here surely lies in the fact that dangerous blood exchanges take place in the process of attempts to make money out of selling blood for therapeutic purposes. These could be simply examples of serious GVHD, especially as the victims are likely to be related and possess very similar blood-groupings.

FINAL COMMENTS/QUESTIONS

In the final analysis, it seems to me that the most pressing need in the AIDS epidemic is education, not only of the undeveloped world, where bad medical practices account for many deaths, but also in the developed world, where well-meaning, sometimes famous, individuals take their information concerning the many aspects of AIDS from the media, and as I have already pointed out, these are largely controlled by commercial interests.

The impression given by the media is that the epidemic can be controlled by use of 'the magic bullets' of so-called retroviral drugs in the undeveloped world. The 'magic bullet' description was applied to the antibiotics such as penicillin, the sulphonamides and streptomycin in the middle years of the last century. These were, and still are, in their various modifications, very useful - often life-saving - today in fighting infections.

AIDS is not in this category of disease. However, the secondary effects of immune insufficiency that render the system unable to counter common agents, easily dealt with by a healthy immune system, can be combatted by treatment of patients with classical antibiotics. It is these antibiotics that need to be promoted, in the present state of our knowledge, rather than treatment with dangerous, expensive so-called anti-retrovirals of doubtful value, which may give the impression of efficacy through acting in a non-specific, inefficient way against secondary infections.

Another area where the public, scientists in distinct but related disciplines (see Foreword), and scientists in general may have been misled is in the surveillance methods that lead to the prediction of the extent of the epidemic. The e-mail exchanges between the CDC and the Perth Group on this point make chilling reading. The replies from the CDC concerning surveillance techniques were flippant and evasive to the point of irresponsibility.

Predictions of the 'HIV' epidemic based on such flimsy premises seem to be reckless and could very well lead to unnecessary and dangerous medical interventions taking place, especially injections of dangerous drugs and blood transfusions, and so causing illnesses diagnosed as AIDS.

Another point that needs to be addressed is whether sero-positivity in women, especially promiscuous ones, is due to allo-antigens from sperm finding their way into the blood-stream, as I have discussed in Chapter Nine in the case of anal sex in gays. Is there in fact self-limiting benign sero-positivity as well as the malignant sort that is diagnostic of AIDS?

Bearing these points in mind, it is important that such lines as I have discussed, however bizarre they may seem at first sight, should be followed up. If I am right about the role of bacteria as vectors of alien DNA (this applies to the various disorders discussed in this book as well as AIDS) then a new approach to vaccines might prove effective as well as being cheap to produce and innocuous. It is above all important that the preconceptions that have hindered AIDS research be put aside. As long as it is necessary to warn research workers that they must not mention any doubts they may harbour about the connection of AIDS and HIV, the nature and relevance of retroviruses or the role of iatrogenesis, or allow the young to hear different views, (a practice discouraged in the US - Lancet 1999) for fear of ridicule and rejection, and even loss of livelihood - we are not likely to advance further in lines of research where these phenomena must be looked in the face and proved true or false on the evidence.

REFERENCES

Brewer, D. D., Brody, S., Drucker E. *et al* (2003) Mounting anomalies in the epidemiology of HIV in Africa : cry the beloved paradigm
Int. J. of STD & AIDS 14 144-147

Gisselquist, D., Potterat, J.J. Brody, S. *et al* (2003) Let it be sexual: how care transmission of AIDS in Africa was ignored
ibid 14 148-161

Guay, L.A., Muske, P.M., Fleming, T. *et al* (1999) Intrapartum and neonatal single-dose nevirapine compared with zidovudine for the prevention of mother-to-child transmission of HIV-1 in Kampala, Uganda: HIVNET 012 randomised trial
Lancet 354 795-802

de Tocqueville, A. (1831) Democracy in America..... as quoted by David Rasnick in Rasnick, D. (2001) Time to Separate State and Science - a talk given at the the International Conference on Science and Democracy - July in Naples Italy.

Hooper, E. (1999) The River: A journey back to the source of HIV and AIDS
Allen Lane The Penguin Press

Ingham, B. (2003) The Wages of Spin. A clear case of communications gone wrong.
John Murray, Albemarle Street, London

Jacques, M. (2004) Democracy isn't working
The Guardian Thursday July 22nd.

Orwell, G. (1976) Nineteen Eighty-Four
Penguin Books in Association with Martin Secker & Warburg

Papadopulos-Eleopulus, E., Turner, V.F., Papadimitriou, J.M. *et al* (2001) Mother to Child Transmission of HIV and its Prevention with AZT and Nevirapine: A Critical Analysis of the Evidence
Riobay Publishing Western Australia 6009

Rasnick, D. (2001) Time to separate State and Science. Talk given at the International Conference on Science and Democracy 20th -21st April Naples Italy
http://www.virusmith.net/aids/data/drstate.htm

Regan, G. (1987) Someone had Blundered...... A Historical Survey of Military Incompetence
B.T. Batsford Ltd. London

Wright, P. (1987) Smallpox Vaccine Triggered AIDS Virus
The Times London

GLOSSARY

AIDS	Acquired Immune Deficiency Syndrome
ALL	Acute Lymphatic Leukaemia
AS	Ankylosing Spondylitis - nearly always associated with HLA B-27
AZT	RT inhibitor also called zidovudine, which is highly toxic and believed by some investigators to cause more harm than good
B-cells	Lymphocytes associated with antibody production
BRU	The initials of the patient in which the first HIV was identified
Caryophanon	Large bacterium found in cow-dung - non-pathogenic; because of its size it is a useful bacterium for the demonstration of bacterial nuclei
CPE	Cytopathogenic (cell-damaging) Effect
CAEV	Caprine arthritis-encephalitis virus - associated with goat arthritis
CEM	A cell-line established in 1966 from lymphocytes from a 4-year old girl with leukaemia.
CD	Crohn's Disease
CD-4	'Helper' T-lymphocytes that recognise MHC Class II fragments. CD-4 counts are used as indicators of the state of the disease in AIDS patients
CD-8	Cytotoxic/Suppressor T-cells - these recognise MHC class I fragments
Cell-lines	Cells growing in culture used for culturing viruses.
CWD	Cell-Wall Deficient forms of bacteria
DNA	Deoxyribonucleic acid
env	The conventional format for the envelope region of retroviruses
E.coli	A rod-shaped single-celled bacterium that is present in the human gut and which is widely used in genetics
ELISA	Enzyme-linked-immunosorbent-assay
Eperithrozoon	An erythrocyte parasite of rodents, now recognised to be a mycoplasma

gag	The classical nomenclature for the core proteins of HIV according to the AIDS mainstream investigators. The 'AIDS antigen' p24 is one of these
GE	Genetic engineering
GGH	Genetic genomic hybridisation
GVHD	Graft Versus Host Disease
GVHR	Graft Versus Host Reaction
H9	A cell-line developed by the Gallo group, very widely used in AIDS research because of the belief that it has developed resistance to HIV
Haemobartonella	A parasite of erythrocytes of rodents
Haemoplasma	The name that replaces *Eperithrozoon* since the latter became recognised as mycoplasmas
HDVT	Human terato carcinoma derived virus
HERV	Human endogenous retroviruses
HIAP	Human Intracisternal Retrovirus - found and identified by the Garry group - H9 was the cell-line used
HIV	Human Immunodeficiency Virus
HLA-B27	The tissue type found in about 92% of patients with AS
HNPCC	Hereditary Non polyposis colorectal cancer
HRV-5	Another retrovirus sequence
HTLV	Human T-cell leukaemia virus
HTRX HRX	Translocation genes
HUT-78	A cell-line derived from a patient with lymphoma - the classic H9 cell-line was derived from it
Iatrogenesis	Disease caused by medical treatment
IBD	Inflammatory Bowel Disease
IDU	Intravenous Drug User

LAI	The initials of the gay male patient from which a vigorous strain of HIV was believed to have been isolated
LFS	Li-Fraumeni Syndrome - a rare hereditable cancer-susceptibility condition
LGE	Laboratory genetic engineering
L-form	This is an early name for cell-wall deficient bacteria. It was derived from the Lister (L) Institute where Klieneberger began her work on them. This term is still sometimes used but it has been largely replaced by CWD
Mycosis fungoides	A T-cell lymphoma
MHC	Major Histocompatibility Complex
MHC-class-I	Encodes for HLA-A HLA-B and HLA-C
MHC-class II	Encodes for DR DW DQ DP
HLA-B27	The Tissue Antigen Associated with some diseases most notably AS
MM	Molecular Mimicry
MCT	Mother to Child Transmission of infective agents
Mycoplasma	Cell-wall-less bacteria, which do not have a walled form
MLL-AF4	A unique gene fusion sequence that indicates that aberrant cells occur during pregnancy
MM	Molecular Mimicry
MMTV	Mouse Mammary Tumour Virus
NGE	Natural Genetic Engineering
NZB	New Zealand Black Mice
NIH-3T3	A culture of mouse embryo fibroblasts
Oscillospira	Large bacterium found in the gut of herbivorous animals
p24	The 'AIDS' antigen
p120	Regarded as an 'AIDS' defining antigen
p53	An important tumour suppressor gene

PAP	Primary Atypical Pneumonia - this condition led to the discovery of *Mycoplasma pneumoniae*, which was the first pathogenic mycoplasma to be discovered in humans
PBC	Primary Biliary Cirrhosis
PBMCs	Peripheral Blood Mononuclear Cells
PCR	Polymerase Chain Reaction
Ph	Philadelphia Chromosome
PPLO	Pleuropneumonia-like Organisms. This term has now been superseded by the name mycoplasma
***Proteus* OX19**	A rod-shaped single-celled bacterium used for the diagnosis of rickettsial infections such as typhus
Pseudomonas	A rod-shaped motile single-celled aquatic bacterium
RA	Rheumatoid Arthritis
Rhizobium	The bacterium associated with root-nodules of legumes, which when infected with the Ti-plasmid causes cancer in the plants
RT	Reverse Transcriptase
RNA	Ribonucleic acid
RSV	Rous Sarcoma Virus
SBE	Sub-bacterial elements - this is yet another expression that means bacteria without the full complement of cell-wall materials
SEM	Scanning Electron-microscopy
SKY	Spectral Karyotyping
SLE	Systemic Lupus Erythematosis
SS	Sjogren's syndrome
Streptobacillus moniliformis	A pleomorphic bacterium that can cause disease, such as rat-bite fever, in humans. In the present context the important point is that it was one of the first demonstrations of L-forms
SWR	Normal white mice used as controls in experiments with NZB

Salmonella typhi	A rod-shaped bacterium that is the causative agent of typhoid fever
Spirillum	Spiral aquatic bacteria that have a readily demonstrable life-cycle
T-cells	Lymphocytes responsible for cell-mediated immunity
STD	Sexually Transmitted Disease
TCR	T-cell receptor - part of the Trimolecular Complex
TEM	Transmission Electron-microscopy
TEL-AML-1	A fusion gene associated with acute lymphoblastic leukaemia
T-DNA	The part of the Ti-plasmid that causes plant cancer
Ti-plasmid	The causative agent of plant cancer
Vitreoscilla	A large gliding bacterium
WB	Western Blot - A technique used for the detection of AIDS antibodies
Weil-Felix Reaction	An agglutination test for the diagnosis of diseases such as typhus
Widal test	A simple agglutination test for the detection of antibodies
Yersinia enterocolitica	Rod-shaped bacterium motile at 22C - shows retrovirus-like elements within the larger elements

APPENDIX ONE

BRIEF NOTES ON SOME AUTOIMMUNE DISEASES

As indicated in Chapter Nine these conditions are difficult to classify, even for the experts. The approaches to them have been diverse and the most important discovery in this area - notably the association of HLA types with certain diseases - was made in studies on the relatively little known condition Ankylosing Spondylytis (AS). Whilst at one time AS was regarded as a variant of RA, the two conditions are now regarded as completely separate since RA is characterised by the presence of rheumatoid factor (RF sero-positivity), which does not occur in AS and related diseases, which are often referred to as the sero-negative Spondyloarthropathies.

The sero-positive ones are sometimes also positive for anti-nuclear antibodies (ANA) and are often referred to as the collagen group. Some of the aspects of the various diseases are described below, together, where feasible, with particular key points *vis a vis* the NGE concept.

RHEUMATOID ARTHRITIS (RA)

This, one of the most well known and commonly occurring autoimmune conditions, is a chronic progressive disease predominantly affecting the joints, which become increasingly more eroded and deformed. There are often systemic manifestations such as the occurrence of nodules, lung and nerve damage and lymphodenopathy. In very simple terms, joint destruction appears to be the result of an attack by the patient's immune system. Immunological activity is demonstrated by the occurrence of lymphocytes, macrophages, immune complexes and complement breakdown products in the joint. One of the earliest changes in the joint is the proliferation of the lining layer cells of the synovium. It affects women mostly and often improves during pregnancy. **It is associated with certain HLA-DR types.**

SYSTEMIC LUPUS ERYTHEMATOSIS (SLE)

SLE has been described as the classic autoimmune disease, since patients suffering from it have abnormalities in almost all parts of their immune system. The onset of the condition can be insidious or can be sudden; exacerbation alternates with remissions and the course of the disease can be variable. It occurs nine times more often in women than in men and is most likely to occur during the child-bearing years, and unlike in RA, there is no improvement during pregnancy. Microchimerism may be a factor in aetiology, which highlights the theme of GVHD that runs through auto/allo immunity.

One third of patients have been shown to be sero-positive for HIV p24 antigen. The MRL/*lpr*/*lpr* mouse model of SLE, produced by extensive inbreeding and back-crossing of a laboratory strain of mice, also manifests anti p24 activity. Kaye (1989) listed thirty one clinical and serological features common to SLE and HIV according to Kion and Hoffman (1991), which suggests a similar type of pathogenesis.

Antibodies to nuclear antigens (ANA) are formed and these are used as diagnostic and prognostic indicators.

PRIMARY BILIARY CIRRHOSIS (PBC)

This is an autoimmune disease of the liver - **30% of patients are p24 sero-positive.**

SCLERODERMA

This is sometimes called 'hard skin' disease, which is the term used to describe the thickening of the skin and its tethering to the sub-cutaneous tissues as well as being the name applied to conditions which also manifest widespread systemic disorders including damage to the heart, lungs, kidneys and intestinal tract. Serious interest in the disease, which was first recognized in the mid nineteenth century, arose when it was included among collagen diseases with SLE Anti-DNA antibodies. **GVHD resemblances. Microchimerism suspected as having a role in pathogenesis.**

SJOGREN'S SYNDROME (SS)

In this disorder dryness of the mouth and/or eyes (sicca syndrome) occurs as a result of immunological activity causing damage to salivary and/or lachrymal glands. Sjogren's original patients also had RA and it is now recognised that whilst the sicca syndrome does occur on its own, *i.e.* primary SS, it is very often accompanied by connective diseases other than RA such as SLE, scleroderma and primary biliary cirrhosis. Patients have an increased risk of the occurrence of B-cell lymphoma. **Resembles GVHD and microchimerism may be involved.**

ANKYLOSING SPONDYLYTIS (AS)

In the present context, **the most important thing about AS is its association with HLA-B27**. AS is an inflammatory disease of the spine, in which fusion of the apophyseal and sacroiliac joints occurs, giving rise to the 'bamboo spine'. It mostly affects young men. It sometimes occurs in association with Inflammatory Bowel Disease (IBD) Ileo-colonoscopy studies have shown 'Crohn's-like' lesions in 57% with active disease.

CROHN'S DISEASE (CD) - AN INFLAMMATORY BOWEL DISEASE (IBD)

This is a disorder of the gut, and any part of it may be affected, but ileocolitis is the commonest type. There is an infiltration of lymphocytes, plasma cells, neutrophils and eosinophils. Granulomas are formed in 70% of patients. Young adults are the main sufferers. **High incidence of HLA B27.**

ULCERATIVE COLITIS (UC) - AN (IBD)

In this condition the affected area is limited to the colon and the inflammation is more superficial than in CD. Both CD and UC may be associated with AS. There is a **high incidence of HLA-B27** in the patients. Arthropathy resembling reactive arthritis may be present.

RHEUMATIC FEVER (RF)

There is a definite connection between Group A streptococci and RF. It occurs 2-3 weeks after a streptococcal throat infection. Damage is caused to the head and the joints, skin and kidneys may be affected. In chronic RF neurological effects in the form of Sydenham's chorea (St. Vitus' dance) may occur. The various symptoms are accompanied by the development of antistreptolysin 0 in the patient's serum. Subsequent re-infection with Group A streptococci, even of a different M type from the original one, may induce a relapse. However, in the case of post infective acute nephritis the streptococcus is the M12 type.

APPENDIX TWO

IS BOVINE SPONGIFORM ENCEPHALOPATHY (BSE) AN AUTOIMMUNE DISEASE?

The most widely accepted theory of the causation of BSE is the prion one (Prusinier 1982). This postulates the existence of an infective agent - virus/prion, which can be transmitted to sheep (scrapie) cows (BSE) and humans (Creutz-Jacob disease CJD). However as Ebringer and his team (Ebringer *et al* 1997) and others have pointed out there are difficulties with this hypothesis. The most conceptually difficult one is the proposition that the agent consists of self-replicating proteins in the absence of DNA. The other point of concern is that the prion sequences are encoded by the host and appear to be a self-protein.

Ebringer *et al* have argued that autoimmunity is the main factor in this type of disease and their evidence is based on the same kinds of evidence they have provided for the molecular mimicry theory of autoimmune disease discussed in this book. Apart from extensive serological evidence, this group has also demonstrated molecular mimicry by the use of space-filling models derived from amino-acid sequence homologies between bovine myelin and prion being comparable to those of bacteria, including *Acinetobacter calcoaceticus* and *Agrobacterium tumefaciens*.

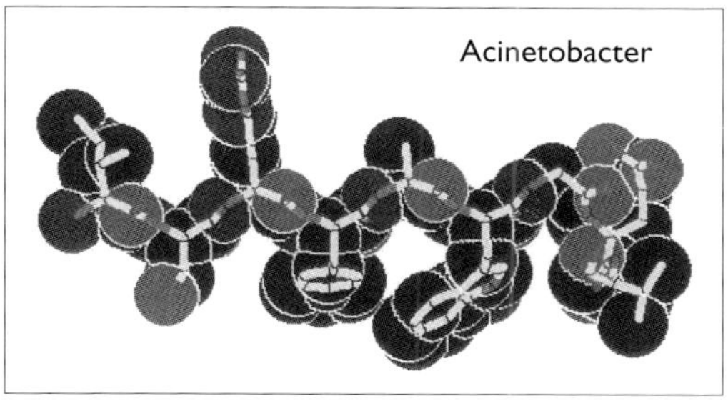

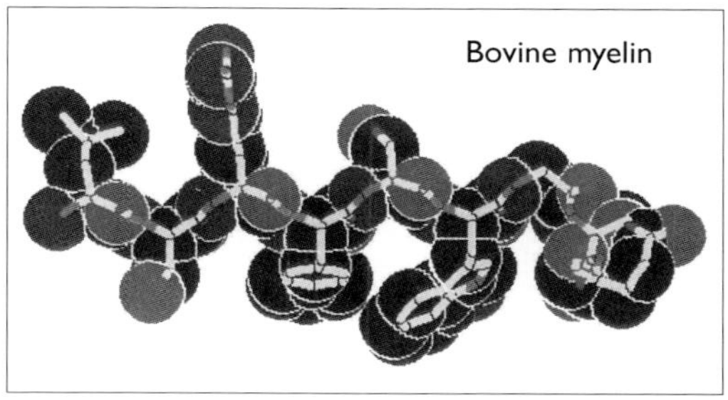

Images by permission of Dr Ebringer

My only personal experience of 'prions' was in collaboration with my colleague Douglas Burdon (Burdon 1989) in studying a replicating agent isolated from the human intestinal tract that had several characteristics in common with the 'unconventional agents associated with CJD and scrapie. It was provisionally named IFDO an acronym for 'ileal fluid dependant organism'.

In brief the agent grew *in vitro* under aerobic and anaerobic conditions both on agar medium and in broth. The colonies on solid medium were dark brown and grew beneath the surface of the agar. IFDO was resistant to steam at 134C, formaldehyde and gluteraldehyde and to some extent ionising radiation. Other similarities to 'slow viruses' were also present. My role in this study was to provide some assistance with electron-microscopy of the agent and this was a disappointing area since it was difficult to identify distinct particles.

As is so often the case in medical research it is difficult to separate cause from effect and in a recent discussion with Douglas Burdon he explained that his belief is that prions have a concealed nucleic acid and that IFDO is an example of such an agent.

If this view is correct I suggest tentatively that the hidden DNA may be present in the episome form and that the molecular mimicry studies of the Ebringer group may give clues as to the composition of the episome DNA that brings about the initial damage to the normal host prions.

REFERENCES

Burdon, D. W. (1989) A novel replicating agent isolated from the human intestinal tract having characteristics shared with Creutzfelt-Jacob and related agents
J.Med Microbiol 29 145-157

Ebringer, A., Pirt, J., Wilson, C. et al. (1997) Bovine spongiform encephalopathy: Is it an autoimmune disease due to bacteria showing molecular mimicry with brain antigens?
Env. Health Perspectives 105: 1172-1174

Prusinier, S. B. (1982) Novel proteinaceous infectious particles cause scrapie
Science 216 136-144

ACKNOWLEDGEMENTS

Colleagues past and present at the University of Birmingham U.K. and attached hospitals

Dr Kenneth A. Bisset; Dr Nancy Laughton; Prof. J.F.D. Shrewsbury; Prof. P.W. Wildy; Dr Barry Cole; Dr L.O.White; Dr Tony Nicholls; Dr Janice Vickerstaff; Dr John Ibbotson; Dr Bobbie Bartlett; Ms Janice Tallack; Ms Ruth Tyler; Ms Hema Chahal; Dr Sue Balmer; Mr John England; Mr David Purdham, Departments of Bacteriology and Medical Microbiology, Medical School, University of Birmingham UK; Ms Sue Dipple and Ms Leslie Tonkin, SEM Facility; Mr C.C. Newton, Department of Electron Physics, TEM Facility; Mr C. Hawkins, Consultant in Rheumatology, Prof. Kenneth Walton and Dr M. Farr, Department of Rheumatology, Queen Elizabeth Hospital Birmingham; Dr Keith Rogers, Children's Hospital Birmingham; Dr Bob Allen, Consultant Gastroenterologist and Dr D. Burdon, Consultant Microbiologist, General Hospital Birmingham; Ms Pauline MacKintosh, Tissue Typing Facility, Birmingham Blood Transfusion Service.

Other co-workers

Prof. Guido Tedeschi - University of Camerino, Italy; Dr E. Alexander-Jackson, University of San Diego, California USA; Prof. John Lawson, University of Clemson, South Carolina; Prof. Alan Ebringer, Kings College, London, UK.

Investigators providing helpful discussions and/or donation of images

Prof. Roni Aloni, University of Tel Aviv, Israel; Dr Lewis Thomas, physician and philosopher - one time head of the Memorial Sloan Kettering Cancer Institute N.Y. City; Prof. Emeritus Etienne de Harven, University of Toronto; Prof. Luc Montagnier, Pasteur Institute, Paris, France; Dr L. Bisset, AIDS Research Switzerland; Mr Julian Bess, SAIC National Cancer Institute - Frederick Cancer Research and Development Centre, Frederick Maryland; Prof. Mel Greaves, Institute of Cancer Research, London UK; Dr Peter Duesberg, University of California, Berkeley, California; Dr Val Turner, Royal Perth Hospital, Western Australia.

Colleagues at Toulouse University providing help and encouragement

Mme Prof. Jacqueline Didier; Prof. Elie Ohayon Professor of Immunologie

Technical support services

David G. Smith, Paul R. Jeffcoat and Ms Anna Essex
Ms Laurie Baker, Science Magazine, Washington DC; Monsieur Alain Warin; Ms June Godfrey

Funding from outside bodies

Arthritis and Rheumatism Council
Back Pain Association
Bicentenary Fund General Hospital Birmingham
British Digestive Foundation
Crohn's in Childhood Research Appeal
Medical Research Council
National Association for Colitis and Crohn's Disease

NOTES